When Medicine Went Mad

Contemporary Issues
in Biomedicine, Ethics, and Society

When Medicine Went Mad: *Bioethics and the Holocaust,*
    edited by *Arthur L. Caplan,* 1992
Compelled Compassion: *Government Intervention in the
    Treatment of Critically Ill Newborns,* edited by *Arthur L.
    Caplan, Robert H. Blank, and Janna C. Merrick,* 1992
New Harvest: *Transplanting Body Parts and Reaping the Benefits,*
    edited by *C. Don Keyes,* 1991
Aging and Ethics, edited by *Nancy S. Jecker,* 1991
Beyond Baby M: *Ethical Issues in New Reproductive Techniques,*
    edited by *Dianne M. Bartels, Reinhard Priester, Dorothy E.
    Vawter, and Arthur L. Caplan,* 1989
Reproductive Laws for the 1990s, edited by *Sherrill Cohen and
    Nadine Taub,* 1989
The Nature of Clinical Ethics, edited by *Barry Hoffmaster,
    Benjamin Freedman, and Gwen Fraser,* 1988
What Is a Person?, edited by *Michael F. Goodman,* 1988
Advocacy in Health Care, edited by *Joan H. Marks,* 1986
Which Babies Shall Live?, edited by *Thomas H. Murray
    and Arthur L. Caplan,* 1985
Alzheimer's Dementia: *Dilemmas in Clinical Research,*
    edited by *Vijaya L. Melnick and Nancy N. Dubler,* 1985
Feeling Good and Doing Better, edited by *Thomas H.
    Murray, Willard Gaylin, and Ruth Macklin,* 1984
Ethics and Animals, edited by *Harlan B. Miller and William H.
    Williams,* 1983
Profits and Professions, edited by *Wade L. Robison,
    Michael S. Pritchard, and Joseph Ellin,* 1983
Visions of Women, edited by *Linda A. Bell,* 1983
Medical Genetics Casebook, by *Colleen Clements,* 1982
Who Decides?, edited by *Nora K. Bell,* 1982
The Custom-Made Child?, edited by *Helen B. Holmes,
    Betty B. Hoskins, and Michael Gross,* 1980
Birth Control and Controlling Birth: *Women-Centered Perspectives,*
    edited by *Helen B. Holmes, Betty B. Hoskins,
    and Michael Gross,* 1980

When Medicine Went Mad

Bioethics and the Holocaust

Edited by

Arthur L. Caplan

*Center for Biomedical Ethics, University of Minnesota,
Minneapolis, Minnesota*

Humana Press ✳ Totowa, New Jersey

portions of the paper by George Annas have been published in

George J. Annas and Michael A. Grodin, editors, *The Nazi Doctors and the Nuremberg Code: Human Rights in Human Experimentation*, Oxford University Press, NY, 1992.

© 1992 The Humana Press Inc.
999 Riverview Dr., Suite 208
Totowa, NJ 07512

Printed in the United States of America

Library of Congress Cataloging in Publication Data

Main entry under title:
When medicine went mad : bioethics and the holocaust / edited by
    Arthur L. Caplan.
        p. cm. — (Contemporary issues in biomedicine, ethics, and
    society)
    Includes bibliographical references (p.) and index.
    ISBN 0-89603-235-3
    1. Human experimentation in medicine—Germany. 2. Medical ethics.
3. World War, 1939–1945—Atrocities. I. Caplan, Arthur L.
II. Series.
R853.H8W54   1992
174'.28—dc20   92-11687
                                                          CIP

Preface

During the past decade, I have had the opportunity of editing and writing many books. None was more difficult to conceive, create, and bring to press than this one.

This book represents the culmination of a long-standing, self-imposed obligation. In 1976, Peter Steinfels, who now reports on religion for *The New York Times,* was a senior colleague of mine at the Hastings Center, the nation's preeminent think tank on issues in bioethics. He had the idea of holding a conference to discuss the implications of the Holocaust for bioethics. Even though I had only recently taken a part time position at the Center, I did not hesitate to let Peter know that I thought his idea was a bad one. I could not see any reason for spending even a day exploring the ethical legacy of a historical event that was so obviously immoral and wrong. What learning or insight could possibly emerge from a discussion of the ethics of genocide, torture, and murder?

Fortunately, wiser heads, namely Daniel Callahan and Willard Gaylin, prevailed, and Peter put together his meeting. No conference has had as profound an impact on me as that one did.

Soon after the half-day conference began, the scholars who were present, including Telford Taylor and Lucy Dawidowicz, made it clear that medicine and science had played crucial roles both in the fostering of Nazi ideology and in implementing the Final Solution. Moreover, it became clear that many of the physicians, public health officials, and scientists who had been involved with the Nazi movement felt no remorse over their activities. They believed they had acted ethically in setting out to sterilize and destroy Jews, Gypsies, homosexuals, and other groups perceived as threats to the racial health of the German nation.

That conference forced me to confront a number of extremely disturbing questions. How could the biomedical establishment of the most sophisticated, technologically advanced nation of its day become so enmeshed with a racist and vile ideology? How could it be that so many doctors and scientists could find moral justifications for their horrible crimes? And, why was it that my own field of bioethics had paid so little attention to the obvious dilemma raised by the reality that Nazi doctors and scientists had grounded their actions in moral language and ethical justifications? If the Holocaust could be defended on ethical grounds then what use is bioethics?

It took more than a decade but, through the efforts of many courageous and generous people, I was able to organize a conference on May 17–19, 1989 at the University of Minnesota to examine the meaning of the Holocaust for Bioethics. The articles collected in this volume represent the results of that meeting.

I am not sure that the authors have answered all of the questions that have troubled me about the need to reconcile my own work in bioethics with the role of biomedicine in the Holocaust. But I am quite certain that this collection of papers goes some way to filling what has been a huge and inexcusable gap in the literature of bioethics.

The organization of this conference and the production of a set of papers on bioethics and the Holocaust was a very, very difficult task. It was next to impossible to find a source of funding for the meeting. Few foundations or donors wanted their name associated with the subject. I would like to extend my deepest appreciation to the Otto Bremer Foundation of St. Paul, Minnesota, the Minneapolis Federation for Jewish Service, the Okinow Foundation, Lieberman Enterprises, Richard and Judith Spiegel, and the College of Liberal Arts, the Medical School, and the Hospital and Clinic of the University of Minnesota for their willingness to support the conference that led to this book. A special debt of gratitude must be extended to Edwin C. (Jack) Whitehead. When it seemed as if the subject matter of bioethics and the Holocaust would prove too controversial for funders he stepped forward and asked his foundation to provide the funds necessary to make this conference happen. Jack Whitehead died early in 1992. I would like to think that he would have taken great pride in seeing this book in print.

Others who played crucial roles in both the conference and the subsequent creation of this book were David Brown, MD, Dean of the University of Minnesota Medical School, who was unstinting in his support, Rabbi Irvin Wise, Morton Ryweck, Louis Newman, John Lavine, Geri Joseph, Bart Galle, Ellen Green, MD, Msgr. James Habiger, Gary J. Stern, and Paul Sand. Robert Pozos, Gisela Konopka, Robert Berger, MD, Charles Carroll, David Lieberman, Robert Proctor, Sam Lieberman, Beth Virnig, and Nancy Segal each played crucial roles in advancing my own thinking about this most difficult subject.

Two of my colleagues here at the Center for Biomedical Ethics at the University of Minnesota, Diane Bartels and Dorothy Vawter, provided important support and intellectual advice and assistance. Toni Knezevich, William Sucha, Patty Vogt, Barbara Higgins, and Lisa Siewart worked long and hard on both the conference and the book. Candace Holmbo went above and beyond the call of duty to make sure that the book became a reality.

Finally, I must single out for special thanks two exceptional people who stuck with me throughout the creation of this book. My father, Sidney, who was among the American troops who liberated the Dachau concentration camp. It was very difficult for him to listen to discussions and debates about the use of data from Nazi medical experiments conducted in the camps, but he never wavered in his support for my belief that the subject had to be examined. And my wife Janet who saw me become at various times agitated, angry, and distraught as I tried to work with the contributors to this volume, think through my own thoughts and feelings about the topics addressed in this book and respond to those who argued that the project should not be done because it touched on subjects that ought to remain taboo. From the time I first decided to do something about the obligation I felt to examine the legacy of the Holocaust for bioethics right up to the appearance of this book she has been my most acute critic while also remaining an unwavering source of support.

Arthur L. Caplan

Contents

The Use of Information from Nazi "Experiments"
The Case of Hypothermia

Medical Killing and Euthanasia:
Then and Now

The Abuse of Medicine
and the Legacy of the Holocaust

Contributors

GEORGE J. ANNAS • *Boston University, Boston, MA*

ROBERT L. BERGER • *Harvard Medical School, Brookline, MA*

ARTHUR L. CAPLAN • *University of Minnesota, Minneapolis, MN*

RONALD CRANFORD • *Hempin County Medical Center, Minneapolis, MN*

BENJAMIN FREEDMAN • *McGill University, Montreal, Quebec, Canada*

VELVL GREENE • *Ben Gurion University Medical School, Beersheva, Israel*

JAY KATZ • *Yale Law School, New Haven, CT*

GISELA KONOPKA • *Minneapolis, MN*

EVA MOZES KOR • *C.A.N.D.L.E.S., Terre Haute, IN*

RUTH MACKLIN • *Albert Einstein College of Medicine, Bronx, NY*

BENNO MULLER-HILL • *University of Cologne, Cologne, FRG*

RICHARD JOHN NEUHAUS • *New York, NY*

ROBERT S. POZOS • *Naval Health Research Center, San Diego, CA*

ROBERT N. PROCTOR • *Pennsylvania State University, University Park, PA*

NANCY SEGAL • *California State University, Fullerton, CA*

WILLIAM SEIDELMAN • *North Hamilton Community Health Center, Hamilton, Canada*

SARA VIGORITO • *C.A.N.D.L.E.S., Cleveland Heights, OH*

xii

Testimonies

Nazi Experiments as Viewed by a Survivor of Mengele's Experiments

Eva Mozes Kor

Introduction

Nothing on this earth can prepare anyone for a place like Auschwitz-Birkenau. One's worse nightmare is mild by comparison to what I had to endure in Mengele' labs. I was just a 9-year-old child who grew up fast, because children who have to face life and death situations are no longer children. I often say that we, the Mengele Twins, are the children without a childhood because when we look back at our wonder years, we remember the huge chimneys, the smell of burned flesh, the shots, the blood taking, the endless tests in Mengele's labs, the rats, lice, and dead bodies that were everywhere.

Although we have received a great deal of attention in the past few years since we, the Mengele Twins, have begun to shed some light on our dark and hidden chapter of the Holocaust, one question was seldom asked, "How did you feel while you were being used as a guinea pig by Josef Mengele?" My answer is that the emotional scars are so deep that only now, more than 40 years later, are we attempting to face our past and come to terms with it. I know that it will always hurt to remember that we were reduced to the lowest form of existence. We were treated like animals—we were his guinea pigs. But it hurts 10 times more today to realize that some American scientists and doctors want to use this data regardless of the unethical manner in which it was obtained; regardless of the pain and suffering paid by the victims. The advocates for the use of the data claim they want to save human lives. It is obnoxious to me that some of the advocates are so magnanimous with other peoples' lives and suffering.

Life in Auschwitz-Birkenau and the Mengele Experiments

In the Spring of 1944, when I arrived in Auschwitz-Birkenau with my family, my twin sister and I were torn away from my mother's arms and we became part of some 1500 sets of twins used by Mengele in his many deadly experiments.

Our day began with roll call at 6 AM, Summer, Winter, rain, or shine; an hour, sometimes two, and one time a whole day—until everyone was accounted for. Then we returned to our barracks where every day we were inspected by Dr. Mengele. He was always accompanied by Dr. Hans König. There were six other people in his entourage. He moved in a nervous pace as he counted us, while snapping his riding stick against his boots. If there were any dead twins in the barracks, he would become very upset.

Three times a week we were taken to the blood lab. There they tied both my arms to restrict the blood flow. In one arm, they gave me shots; from the other they took blood, lots of blood—at least two vials and often more. On a few occasions, I saw twins faint from loss of blood. They wanted to learn how much blood we could lose and still survive.

Once a week we were taken to the shower room, given a bar of soap, and our clothes were disinfected in a fruitless effort to rid us of lice; we were covered from head to toe. Three times a week we were taken (always accompanied by an SS guard) to the Auschwitz I labs for experiments. These would last from 8–10 hours. They would strip us naked and put a group of us, all children, in a big room. Every part of our body was measured, photographed, marked, and compared to charts. Every movement we made was noted. I felt like a piece of meat. (They had my body but not my spirit, which dreamed of freedom.) These experiments were emotionally very difficult to deal with, but the deadly ones were done in the blood lab.

In early July, 1944, I was injected with some kind of a germ. By evening I became very ill. I had a very high fever and I was trembling. I could hardly move or think. On my next visit to the blood lab, the doctors did not tie my arms, as usual, but took my temperature. I was desperately trying to hide the fact that I was ill because there was a rumor that no one came back from the hospital alive. My fever was very high and I was sent to the hospital. Mengele came to see me twice a day with four other doctors. They checked my fever chart but never examined me. I was given no food, no water, no medication. I remember one of the doctors said sarcastically, "Too bad she has only two weeks to live," but I was determined to get well and be reunited with my twin sister, Miriam. I made a silent pledge to fight with all my being to survive. Today I know that if I would have died, Mengele would have killed my twin sister with a phenol shot to the heart and then performed autopsies on our bodies, comparing my diseased organs with Miriam's. I remember waking up on the barrack floor, fading in and out of consciousness, and saying to myself, "I must survive!" I was crawling to the other end, to reach a faucet with water. After two weeks my fever broke and I was reunited with Miriam. Six months later, on January 27, 1945, we were liberated in Auschwitz by the Russian army.

Life After Liberation

Coping with Trauma and Disease

After liberation, I thought that my problems would be over, but that was not true. We spent over nine months in three Displaced Persons (DP) camps, in the Soviet Union. In late September we returned home. No one else from our family survived. For those terrible 10 months in camp I had one sentence that I kept saying everyday, "Someday soon, I will be free and I will go home." The picture of home that I dreamed about was: mother, father, two older sisters, and us, the twins. This dream never came true; it is forever ever buried in the ashes of Auschwitz-Birkenau.

The first year back from camp (we were living with an aunt in Rumania) we were covered with boils and blisters. The doctors told us that we were suffering from malnutrition. In May of 1946, we went to the first Memorial Service for the Holocaust. The rabbi asked us to bring any soap we might have from the death camps for a burial ceremony. At that time I discovered that the soap that I had been washing with for two years was made out of human fat. I began having nightmares that the soap I had been using was made out of my own parents. These nightmares plagued me for four years, not ceasing until I emigrated to Israel in June, 1950.

In 1960, I married an American tourist and came to live in Terre Haute, Indiana. Miriam was already married and she just had her first baby. Then she became very ill with kidney problems. After many tests, they found that her kidneys were the size of a very young child's and, overburdened by her pregnancy, they could not function adequately.

By 1987 she had become so ill that the doctor said that she needed a kidney transplant in order to survive. On November 16, 1987, I donated her my left kidney. I saved her life in Auschwitz, I could not let her die now. We were a perfect match because we are identical twins. She was fine for one year. Then she developed cancer polyps. According to her doctors, this resulted from the anti-rejection medication that combined with some strange substances that were already in her body. Her doctors are puzzled by it. If we could find our files from Auschwitz it might help the doctors find a cure for her, and for many other Mengele twins who suffer incurable mysterious diseases.

The Nazi Data

What Should Be Done?

Regarding the Nazi data: I am appalled by anyone who seemingly is justifying the means by using the results of the Nazi experiments. In Auschwitz we were treated like a commodity; the hair was used for mattresses; the fat was used for soap; the skin for lampshades; the gold collected from the teeth of the dead went into the Nazi treasury, and many of us were used as guinea pigs. Today some doctors want to use the only thing left by these victims. They are like vultures waiting for the corpses to cool so they could devour every consumable part. To use the Nazi data is obscene and sick. One can always rationalize that it would save human lives, the question should be asked, at what cost?

American scientists and doctors are regarded as having moral and ethical values and are held in very high esteem in the world. To declare the use of the Nazi data ethical, as some of the American scientists and doctors advocate, would open a Pandora's box and could become an excuse for any of the Ayatollahs, Kadafis, Stroessners, and Mengeles of the world to create similar circumstances whereby anyone could be used as their guinea pig.

In the case of the Mengele Twins, copies of the data should be given to those twins who are still alive. The data of the victims who are dead should be shredded and placed in a transparent monument, as evidence that they exist, but cannot be used. It should be a lesson to the world that human dignity and human life are more important than any advance in science or medicine.

I, Eva Mozes Kor, a survivor of the Nazi medical and genetic experiments, appeal to all scientists and doctors to make a pledge to do the following things:

1. Take a moral commitment never to violate anyone's human rights and human dignity.

2. To promote a universal idea that says; "Treat the subjects of your experiments in the manner that you would want to be treated if you were in their place."
3. To do your scientific work, but please, never stop being a human being. The moment you do, you are becoming a scientist for the sake of science alone, and you are becoming the Mengele of today.

From: *When Medicine Went Mad* Ed.: A. Caplan
©1992 The Humana Press Inc.

A Profile of Nazi Medicine

The Nazi Doctor—His Methods and Goals

Sara Seiler Vigorito

The challenge has caught up with us. Should we align ourselves with the practices of Nazi scientists and physicians or should we draw a strict division between what was then and what is now. How can we decide what is ethical, if anything, when using tainted Nazi data? In order to come to any kind of clear conclusion about this dilemna, we need to start at the beginning and create a clear focus and direction.

The words data, experimentation, records, physicians, scientists, and informed consent, bring to mind clearly written accurate records; experiments conducted on animals or at least with informed consent on human beings; people who are generally honest and reliable led by a strong desire to improve and extend human life, and a quiet, respectable exchange or agreement between doctor/scientist and patient. In Nazi Germany, none of these were ever the case.

The Nazi doctor was a physician turned inside out. Rather than striving to extend human life, the Nazi doctor and scientist experimented and schemed for the quickest and most efficient method to wisk out a human life. Benzine, gasoline, hydrogen proxide, evipan, prussic acid (cyanide), chloroform, and air were all substances injected into the veins of innocent concentration camp victims to accomplish their murder. Phenol injected directly into the heart ventricle came to be the most "inexpensive, easy to use, and absolutely effective method" of murder by lethal injection used by the Nazi doctors. In order to come to this conclusion, hundreds of victims were murdered and the results were recorded. These data weres not records of life-saving methods, rather they are a record of how the most efficient method of murdering human beings was devised in the name of medical science.

There was an interest among Nazi doctors to discover the secret of multiple births. If the Nazi scientists could acquire this knowledge, the Aryan Uebermensch could be multiplied at double the natural rate and world conquest would be more imminent. Doctor Josef Mengele, Chief Medical Officer of Auschwitz-Birkenau Concentration Camp, prided himself on his research on twins. The twins were usually children. I was one of these children and I spent a year in a wooden cage in Mengele's private laboratory. The data recorded was obtained through human torture that frequently caused the death of the twins involved and almost always had an end result of murder. Here, the Nazi scientist/physician had as his goal the furthering of the life of a select group that would then enslave or murder the rest of humanity. The victims were considered nothing other than "items for experimentation, to be disposed of when the information needed was recorded." All this at the expense of the murder of innocent children.

Since Nazi doctors had so many human beings at their disposal, they also became involved in disease experimentation. Typhus, tuberculosis, and syphilis to name a few, were injected into victims to study the progress of the disease. Patients were not treated for the disease. Rather, they were observed, data were recorded, the victims were murdered, an autopsy was performed to study the internal effects of the disease, more data were recorded, and the victim's body was exterminated. Nazi doctors again studied disease and recorded data for the benefit of the select few (Aryans), at the expense of murder. Informed consent was unheard of in Nazi concentration camps.

It is most important to realize that these Nazi physicians or scientists were not monsters or madmen. The Nazi doctor did not have any physical or immediately recognizable distinction that would set him apart from our family doctor. After my sister and I were selected by Mengele for his experiments on twins and diseases, we had almost daily contact with him. It is from this perspective that I hope to include here a description of the nature of the Nazi doctor and his "experiments." In this way, I hope to give the modern scientist/physician a clearer view of the dangers in attitudes involved in scientific research. All we need to do is reverse our priorities, leaving human life as secondary, superceded by science and progress. In doing this, the scientist becomes a researcher working in the shadow of Mengele and his Nazi counterparts. Thus, each of us has within us the potential to become a "Nazi" doctor. My hope is that this personality profile will become a deterrent in bringing this about.

Mengele loved precision and order and these rated above everything else. He would not tolerate carelessness and he demanded respect from his colleagues and "patient" victims. He was extremely intelligent and although his victims feared him, he was never thought of as a monster. Rather, it was the depth of his intellect twisted into a science of human destruction that we, even the youngest of his victims, feared most. Mengele was a quiet man who expressed his wishes clearly and with very few words. He seldom raised his voice but carried out displeasures by efficiently fulfilling the consequences. Mengele did not deal with emotions or feelings. There were times when he abruptly left the room when confronted with the wailing of child victims...almost as if he feared that he might be moved with pity and discontinue his experiments. He would not return until the next day...when he conducted his torturous experiments. Intermingled with the above characteristics are also those that make up a good doctor or scientist. However, unlike the ethical physician/scientist, the Nazi scientist did not have the preservation of human life and relief of suffering as his ultimate goal. "Somehow he had become trapped in himself and in his own selfish gains." To him, "efficiency" and "science for its own sake" had become the alpha and the omega, and he had slipped over the edge and made science his god. Human life became expendable through the process of dehumanization; i.e., selected groups of human beings were considered inferior and subhuman, subsequently...expendable. Mengele's efficiency permitted no waste. He wasted no time on acquiring consent from his victims nor on emotions by demonstrating compassion. Experiments were carried out without anesthesia or pain relievers that would have been wasteful and inefficient. Subsequently, the "experiments" conducted by the Nazi doctor were no longer experiments as we understand experiment today—they were methods of nothing less than human torture. These Nazi "experiments" did not include concern in any way for the life or suffering of its victims. They were carried out efficiently for the sole benefit of science, leaving murder and human torture in their path. For example:

> Dr. Mengele approaches a wooden cage in which two small children are imprisoned. He points to one of the children and orders that the child be brought into the examining room. The child is layed onto the examining table naked. Its mouth is gagged and eyes are blindfolded. Assistants hold the child down onto the table on each side. The doctor steps forward with his scalpel and makes a long incision into the child's left leg along the tibia. He then begins to take scrapings from the bone. When he is finished, the leg is bound up and the child is returned to the cage...nothing is given for pain.*

When the victim did not cooperate with the doctor, he often paid with his life or was subjected to torture that resulted in murder. All this was carried out without much ado from the doctor. He was very matter-of-fact, very efficient; he just gave orders. The Nazi doctor frequently had a family and when his day's work was done, he went home to his wife and children. He was a father and a husband.

*from: Sara Vigorito's personal memoirs.

After having provided this brief profile of the Nazi doctor, his value system, and method of his "experimentation," should the data resulting from the torture of his victims be reused? My response is that the scientist who reuses these data aligns himself with the values and methods of the Nazi scientists/doctors by extending their work into contemporary research, thereby giving it credibility and sanction. He too is saying first and foremost, "for the sake of science" and for the sake of "progress," ignoring the case for humanity. Some say that the Nazi medical data should be available in the event that it could save a human life. History has yet to prove that the nature of man is such that after using tainted data to save "one human life," he would then reject it for further use. The data consist of documentations of "stolen" human lives. To draw profit from stolen goods is to incorporate with the thief.

We have, at times, bargained with the evil tactics of other nations. For example, we returned Iranian terrorists to Iran to free the lives of American hostages. Our willingness to bargain in this way became a profitable enterprise for the Iranians and thereby endangered the lives of all Americans in Iran. Our willingness to bargain with Nazi evil and make use of its results will endanger human lives and dignity by placing them second to the conquest of "science." Science and medicine are designed to exist for the benefit of humankind, but they can only maintain this dignity and respectability when they are the "servant" of human life and well-being. Any compromise thereof turns science into a trade of egotism and bigotry.

From: *When Medicine Went Mad* Ed.: A. Caplan
©1992 The Humana Press Inc.

The Meaning of the Holocaust for Bioethics

Gisela Konopka

I speak not only as a victim, but as an active resister to the Nazis. I was 23 years old and living in Hamburg, Germany when the Nazis came to power. Long before that time, even all through my adolescence, I was imbued with the idea that every human being must fight injustice wherever it occurs. Since 1933, I have been an anti-Nazi fighter in Germany, Austria, and France. I spent a short time in a concentration camp near Hamburg and in a prison in Vienna. In this framework of experience I will now relate to the subject of this book.

I want to make it clear first that Nazi persecutions started the moment they came to power in 1933, six years before what has become known as the Holocaust. There were almost immediately restrictive laws for Jews. Jewish professors were dismissed. Anyone who expressed disagreement with Nazi thinking—if found out or denounced—was imprisoned. Only those who did not want to know did not know. Yet all knew fear.

Racism Was at the Core of Nazi Ideology

Nazi persecution of the Jews was not a religious persecution, it was a racial persecution, racism in its worst form. It was based on two premises on which all racism is based:

(1) that there is a race that is superior to all others. In the case of the Nazis, it was the Germanic one; (2) that anyone who disagrees with that idea becomes part of the inferior race. Those dissenters are frequently forgotten. They included courageous Germans and Jews.

From those two premises, according to the Nazis, it followed that people of inferior races (that included Gypsies and Poles and anyone who did not agree with the ideology of Germanic superiority) must be eliminated and destroyed. Also, because of their own sense of inferiority and their hate toward anybody who had succeeded in one form or another, killing was not enough. Torture and demeaning had to be added. Hate of the Jews was especially strong because of a century-old history, almost a tradition, in Europe of persecution of Jews and because of a fear of anyone who was a "stranger," who had different customs than the rest of society. Centuries ago, persecution of Jews was based on religion. This was definitely not the case under the Nazis. They persecuted Jews because of their so-called "racial inferiority" which, according to the Nazis, meant that Jews had to be erased from the earth.

The Dehumanization of Human Beings

The medical experiments done in the concentration camps were in no way scientific undertakings. They were sadistic, depersonalized attacks disguised as science. Almost all the medical so-called experiments, including those of freezing people to death, were done without the use of anesthetics. In no way would this make them more acceptable. This is only an additional indication that this was not a scientific undertaking. Also, why was there such an emphasis on so-called scientific experiments related to the genitalia? All theories of racial hatred include preoccupation with sex, implying that members of any so-called inferior race need to be feared because of their intent to rape the so-called beautiful, superior race! Early Nazi laws that forbade women under 45 years of age to serve in a Jewish household that included a male member, were based on this insulting nonsense. To the Nazis, those people were not persons. There were no "good intentions" as Richard Neuhaus implies. The "Volk" and social hygiene ideologies were screens and falsehoods. "All for the Volk" was not an ideology. It was a rationalization of sadistic impulses.

I remember that early in 1933 (I cannot remember the occasion), one young Nazi doctor inoculated one person after another, including myself, with the same needle without sterilizing it. In my presence someone mentioned the need for clean needles to him. He laughed and said, "For those? Who cares!"

Using Information from Nazi Research

In the concentration camp I saw a man hunted to death by making him run, fall down, get up, and run again until the blood spurted out of his mouth. Perhaps someone could develop "scientific" data on how long it takes for a lung to burst!

By the way, all those immense discoveries in the hypothermia data do not seem so great to me. I knew already as a teenager (before the Nazis) that to drink alcohol and fall asleep in the snow may bring death.

I consider it inexcusable to dignify those murderers with the word "scientist" or dignify what they did with the word "research." Research with people must recognize the human being as valuable. We do expect informed consent even if we use placebos. To the Nazis, people were only material objects. Himmler used the word "Menschenmaterial." There was torture, and especially degradation. That proves that this was not well meant or cool science. Therefore, as one answer to the questions Arthur Caplan raised in the beginning of the conference: No dignity should be afforded to the data or to those who produced them. The data should be thrown to the wind and forgotten. No torture permits someone else's life to be saved. We can make our own discoveries without offending humanity.

Lessons from the Holocaust

Now to some additional thinking about what we have
learned. We have to always remember a very basic principle,
that science in itself is valueless and so is technology. In the
use of both in a world inhabited by people, human ethics and
values must enter.

Robert Proctor and others speak of physicians as scientists. They are not. They are professionals building part of
their knowledge on science, part on experience, and part on
their own good judgment. Today when patients are prepared
for surgery they rightfully sign a statement that indicates
the acknowledgment that medicine is not an exact science.
That does not diminish that great profession. It only means
that ethics—as in all applied professions—become indispens-
able. I am quoting from Maxwell Anderson:

> "....science is completely impartial. It doesn't give a
> damn which way to go. It can invent the atom bomb
> but it can't tell you whether to use it or not. Science is
> like—well, it's like a flashlight in a totally dark room
> measuring two billion light years across—and with
> walls that shift away from you as you go toward them.
> The flash can show you where your feet are on the
> floor; it can show you the furniture or the people close
> by; but as for which direction you should take in that
> endless room it can tell you nothing."[2]

Science and technology do not equal humanity. This was
Einstein's dilemma and he was very aware of it. We may disagree in application to individual cases and situations, but I
think we can crystallize two basic values or measuring sticks
that are absolute and should be used at any time. They are
the importance of the dignity of each individual regardless
of his/her origin, and so forth, and the responsibility of people
for each other.

All over the world those values were expressed by many
great religions and individuals, even though they differed

sometimes on the origin of those values. The Judeo-Christian injunction says, "Love thy neighbor like thyself." The Humanist postulates, "All men are brothers." "The whole of humanity shall be a united people" (Ramakrishna, India's religious reformer). "Wound no others. Do no one injury by thought or deed, utter no word to pain thy fellow creatures" (the Code of Manu-Hindu). "Harm no living thing" (Buddhist). "Never do to others what you would not like them to do to you" (Confucius). "The moral law within you" (Kant).

The Holocaust has given us a stern warning. As a historian, I may add that there were other such warnings too. Let us not forget the lynching and torturing of slaves. Those have shown what it means when we forget basic human values. In each case, whatever we do we have to assess whether we are violating the principle of the value of each human being, and our responsibility for each other.

Also, any arguments for the use of Nazi data or practice that use "others did this too" should be rejected. I have heard too often, "The Americans, the English, and so on did this too." No lynching or racist theories in the US excuse any torture under the Nazis. Nor does any tortures during the Holocaust excuse a single discrimination or racial slur in the US or anywhere else in the world.

Finally, regarding the responsibility of intellectuals, then and now: It shames me to think that members of a university would want to use bogus knowledge gained under such inhumane circumstances. To me, universities and a free press are the most important safeguards of a free society. If they fall, we may lose too much. I know that they can be corrupted as they were in Germany. Not every one of the professors at the German universities agreed with the Nazis, but too many were silent. Those who worked actively with them and did the medical experiments were criminals with so-called clean hands, fine titles, and good employment. Money is unfortunately an effective incentive to commit crimes. Unfortunately, sharp intellects have the capacity to find rationalizations for atrocities. Solzhenitsyn wrote:

"What is the most precious thing in the world? Not to participate in injustices. They are stronger than you. They have existed in the past and they will exist in the future. But let them not come about through you."[3]

Too easily one can be swayed by personal ambition and the comfort that surrounds people in university settings to let things just happen. Greed and arrogance can be used to hurt others. We need people with courage, with no arrogance because of their position, their intelligence, their race, or whatever, to act according to a conscience. The Reverend Michael Scott, active in the fight against Apartheid in South Africa, said it better than I can say it:

"If you believe in the dignity of men, you must uphold it wherever it is being disregarded."

That is what we learn from the Holocaust.

From: *When Medicine Went Mad* Ed.: A. Caplan
©1992 The Humana Press Inc.

Medicine, Bioethics, and Nazism

Nazi Biomedical Policies[1]

Robert N. Proctor

For many historians and philosophers of science, the assumption for most of this century has been either that science is *inherently democratic* (that is, it depends on and contributes to democratic political formations), or that it is *apolitical*, and that the politicization of science implies its destruction. Science, in this view, must have only itself as a goal and a guide; science in the service of "interests" is no longer science. Implicit in this model is the view that science cannot flourish in a society that requires (asks?) science to serve interests other than itself. There is a politics implicit in this judgment: Namely, that science grows only on the soil of democracy and that social forces hostile to democracy will be hostile to science. Such a view holds that the fate of science in a totalitarian regime is that it will be suppressed; the possibility that science (or scientists) might contribute to fascist movements is ruled out of court.

Given such a view, it is not hard to understand why philosophers have generally failed to come to grips with science under fascism: Philosophers have generally assumed that there could not have been anything worthy of the name science under the Nazis. Indeed, as one philosopher in the 1960s put it, National Socialism "had hardly sufficient logical coherence to deserve the name of ideology."[2]

What I want to argue here, however, is that such a view is not borne out when we look at the experience of science

23

under National Socialism. Although it is true that certain
fields, such as theoretical physics, did suffer—in most senses
of that term—it is also true that others, such as anthropology or "genetic pathology," actually flourished—in a limited
sense of that term.[3]

As we shall see, biomedical scientists played an active
and leading role in the initiation, administration, and execution of each of the major Nazi racial programs. In this sense,
science (and especially biomedical science) under the Nazis
cannot simply be seen in terms of an essentially passive and
apolitical scientific community responding to external political forces. This model of science as passive and apolitical in
the face of Nazi racial politics underestimates the extent to
which political initiatives arose from within the scientific
community, and the extent to which science and technology
were integral parts of the Nazi program. It is a mistake, in
other words, to view the relation of science and government
in this period as essentially one of hostility. Certain sciences
were suppressed, but others did quite well.[4]

But I also want to argue that it is wrong to focus exclusively on science or technology as the guilty party in Nazi
crime. The technologies used by Nazi ideologues were shaped
by political priorities, and nothing inherent in instrumental
logic or the technological process brought about these crimes.
Nazi science represents the triumph of a particular kind of
science but not of science in general. In fact, it was ultimately
a political movement—the seizure of state power by the Nazi
party—that allowed forces hostile to life and liberty to be
unleashed within the scientific community.

Biomedicine in the Nazi Racial State

The kind of science I want to focus on is what was known
as "racial hygiene." At the end of the 19th century, German
Social Darwinists, fearing a general "degeneration" of the
human race, set about to establish a new kind of hygiene—a
racial hygiene (*Rassenhygiene*)—that would turn the attention of physicians away from the individual or the environ-

ment, toward the human "germ plasm." In the eyes of its founders (Alfred Ploetz and Wilhelm Schallmayer), racial hygiene was supposed to complement personal and social hygiene; racial hygiene would provide long-run, preventive medicine for the German germ plasm by combatting the disproportionate breeding of "inferiors," the celibacy of the upper classes, and the threat posed by feminists to the reproductive performance of the family.

In 1918, Hermann W. Siemens identified racial hygiene as "a political program that stands above all parties"; racial hygiene was based on "the facts of inheritance and variability." Inheritance taught that "man owes the essential part of his character, good or bad, physical or spiritual, to his genetic material (*Erbmasse*)." Variability taught that "men differ substantially in their genetic value (*Erbwert*)," and that "there are men who are genetically fit, and men who are genetically unfit." It followed, Siemens argued, that if those who are fit breed less than those who are inferior, the quality of the race will decline. The goal of a "positive racial hygiene" was to ensure that the fit leave more offspring than the unfit. If we fail in this, "all other earthly strivings will be in vain." More specifically, Germany will collapse in the face of an "Asiatic triumph."[5]

Interestingly, the early racial hygiene movement was primarily nationalistic and meritocratic more than it was antisemitic or Nordic supremacist. Eugenicists worried more about the indiscriminate use of birth control (by the "fit") and the provision of inexpensive medical care (to the "unfit"), than about the breeding of superior with inferior races, or many of the other themes we associate with the Nazis. Antisemitism played a relatively minor role in early racial hygiene. In fact, for Ploetz, father of the German movement (his 1895 treatise, in which he coined the term *Rassenhygiene* served as the most important early book on this topic), Jews were to be classed along with the Nordics as one of the superior, cultured races of the world.[6]

By the mid-1920s, however, this had changed, and the right-wing faction of racial hygiene had merged with National Socialism. The conservative, antisemitic J. F. Lehmann

Verlag took over publication of the *Archiv für Rassen- und Gesellschaftsbiologie* (the main racial hygiene journal) shortly after the war, and Nazi ideologues began to incorporate eugenics rhetoric into their discourse.

Traditionally, historians and philosophers have stressed the romantic origins of National Socialism: the links to German idealism, the nihilism of Nietzsche, or the Aryan supremist ideology of Gobineau, Chamberlain, and Lapouge. Biology (and especially biologism[7]), however, also played an important role in Nazi ideology. Fritz Lenz, for example (one of Germany's most prominent racial hygienists), praised Hitler in 1930 as "the first politician of truly great import who has taken racial hygiene as a serious element of state policy." Hitler himself was lauded as the "great doctor of the German people"; he once called his revolution "the final step in the overcoming of historicism and the recognition of purely biological values."

Biological imagery was important in Nazi literature in several ways. *SS* journals spoke of the need for "selection" to replace "counter-selection," borrowing their language directly from the social Darwinian rhetoric of the racial hygienists. Nazi leaders commonly referred to National Socialism as *applied biology*; indeed it was Lenz who originally coined this phrase in the 1931 edition of his widely read textbook on human genetics.[8]

The Nazi state was itself supposed to be *biologisch,* or organic, in two separate senses: in its suppression of dissent (the organic body does not tolerate one part battling with another) and in its emphasis on natural modes of living. Nature and the natural mode of living were highly prized by Nazi philosophers: Women were not supposed to wear make-up, and legislation was enacted to protect endangered species. Hitler, as we know, was a vegetarian and did not smoke or drink, nor would he allow anyone to do so in his presence. One of the period's most powerful physicians, Hans Reiter declared the Nazi state "first in the world," judged by the organic views of its leaders.

Given the importance of biology in Nazi discourse, it is not surprising that doctors were among those most strongly attracted to the Nazi movement. In 1929, a number of physicians formed the National Socialist Physicians League to coordinate Nazi medical policy and purify the German medical community of "Jewish Bolshevism." The organization was an immediate success, with nearly 3,000 doctors representing 6% of the entire profession joining the League by January 1933—that is, *before* the rise of Hitler to power. Doctors, in fact, joined the Nazi Party earlier and in greater numbers than any other professional group. By 1942, more than 38,000 doctors had joined the Nazi Party, nearly half of all doctors in the country. In 1937, doctors were represented in the *SS* seven times more often than was the average for the employed male population; doctors assumed leading positions in German government and universities.

Pawns or Pioneers?

One often hears that National Socialists distorted science, that doctors perhaps cooperated more with the Nazi regime than they should have, but that by 1933, as one emigré said, it was too late, and scientists had no alternative but to cooperate or flee. There is certainly some truth in this, but I think it misses the more important point that medical scientists were the ones who invented racial hygiene in the first place. Many of the 20-odd university institutes for racial science and racial hygiene were established at German universities before the Nazi rise to power, and by 1932, it is fair to say that racial hygiene had become a scientific orthodoxy in the German medical community. Racial hygiene was taught in the medical faculties of most German universities; racial hygiene was the subject of special lectures and seminars. The major expansion in this department occurs before Hitler comes to power; most of the dozen or so journals of racial hygiene, for example, were established long before the triumph of National Socialism.

Racial hygiene was recognized as the primary research goal of two separate institutes of the prestigious Kaiser Wilhelm Gesellschaft: the Kaiser Wilhelm Institute for Anthropology in Berlin (1927–1945), directed by Eugen Fischer, and the Kaiser Wilhelm Institute for Genealogy in Munich (1919–1945), directed by psychiatrist Ernst Rüdin. Both institutes performed research in the fields of criminal biology, genetic pathology, and what we today would call human genetics. They also helped train SS physicians construct the "genetic registries" later used to round up Jews and Gypsies. Twin studies were among the leading preoccupations of these and other racial hygiene institutes. The purpose was to sort out the relative influence of nature and nurture in human character and institutions. This was to become one of the major priorities of Nazi medical research. In 1939, Interior Minister Wilhelm Frick ordered all twins born in the Reich to be registered with Public Health Offices for purposes of genetic research.

The Kaiser Wilhelm Institutes for racial hygiene were funded very well. In 1935, the Rüdin Institute alone received 300,000 RM, more than the Kaiser Wilhelm Institutes for Physics and Chemistry combined. The largest such institution, however, was Otmar von Verschuer's Frankfurt Institute for Racial Hygiene. This institute had 67 rooms and several laboratories; this was where Josef Mengele did his doctoral research on the genetics of cleft palate, working under Verschuer. Mengele was also appointed assistant to Verschuer, and provided "experimental materials" to the Institute (including eyes, blood, and other body parts) from Auschwitz as part of a study on the racial specificity of blood types (funded by the Deutsche Forschungsgemeinschaft). This, I should note, was one of the reasons blood groups were so actively studied in the 1930s. When Otto Reche founded the German Society for Blood Group Research in 1926, one of the main reasons he gave for this was to see if he could find a reliable means of distinguishing various races in the test tube.

Scientists, in other words, were not simply pawns in the hands of Nazi officials. But without a strong state to back them, racial hygiene was relatively impotent. It was not until 1933 and the triumph of Hitlerian fascism that the programs of the preNazi period gained the support of officials willing to move aggressively in this area.

The Sterilization Law

What were the practical results of Nazi racial hygiene? Three main programs—the Sterilization Law, the Nuremberg Laws, and the euthanasia operation—formed the heart of the Nazi program of medicalized, "racial cleansing." These (and especially the euthanasia program) were the programs that cleared the path for subsequent efforts to eliminate entire peoples from European soil.

On July 14, 1933, the Nazi government passed the Law for the Prevention of Genetically Diseased Offspring, or Sterilization Law, allowing the forcible sterilization of anyone suffering from genetically determined illnesses, including feeble-mindedness, schizophrenia, manic depressive insanity, genetic epilepsy, Huntington's chorea, genetic blindness, deafness, or severe alcoholism. The measure was drawn up after a series of meetings by several of Germany's leading racial hygienists, including Fritz Lenz, Alfred Ploetz, Ernst Rüdin, Heinrich Himmler (who had been active in breeding chickens prior to 1933), Gerhard Wagner (Führer of the National Socialist Physicians' League), and Fritz Thyssen, the industrialist.

In 1934, 181 Genetic Health Courts and Appellate Genetic Health Courts were established throughout Germany to adjudicate the Sterilization Law. The courts were usually attached to local civil courts and presided over by two doctors and a lawyer, one of whom had to be an expert on "genetic pathology." According to the provisions of the law, doctors were required to register every case of genetic illness known to them; physicians could be fined 150 RM for failing to register any genetic defective. Physicians were also required to undergo training in "genetic pathology" at one of the numerous racial institutes established throughout the country. Also in 1934, the German Medical Association founded a journal, *Der Erbarzt* (The Genetic Doctor), to help physicians determine who should be sterilized; the journal also described the latest sterilization techniques.

Estimates of the total number of people sterilized in Germany range from 350,000 to 400,000. In some areas, more than 1% of the total population was sterilized. Compared with the demands of some racial hygienists this was relatively modest. Lenz, for example, had argued that as many as 10–15% of the entire population were defective and ought to be sterilized.

As a consequence of the law, sterilization research and engineering rapidly became one of the largest medical industries. Medical supply companies (such as Schering) designed sterilization equipment; medical students wrote more than 180 doctoral theses exploring the criteria, methods, and consequences of sterilization. There were obvious incentives for developing more rapid sterilization techniques, especially for women, for whom the standard procedure of tying the tubes could involve a hospital stay of more than a week. The most important of these techniques was the development of "operationless" sterilization involving scarification of the fallopian tubes through injections of supercooled carbon dioxide. In 1943, the gynecologist Clauberg announced to Himmler that using such a technique and with a staff of 10 men, he could sterilize as many as 1,000 women a day. Scarification was not the only new technique developed. According to one study, 12% of all sterilizations were performed with X-rays, a technique also used in the US during this period.

I should also mention that it was the US that provided the most important model for German sterilization laws.[9] By the late 1920s, 15,000 individuals had been sterilized in the US—most while incarcerated in prisons or homes for the mentally ill. Nearly half of these took place in California—

most of the others in northern states (not, as one might have expected, in the South). German racial hygienists throughout the Weimar period expressed their envy of American achievements in this area, warning that unless the Germans made progress in this field, America would become the world's racial leader.

Racial Medicine: The Control of Women

Racial domination and the elimination of the weak and unproductive were not the only forms of oppression in the Nazi regime. One aspect of Nazi ideology that has come under increasing scrutiny in recent years is the masculine and machismo nature of that ideology. Of the 2.5 million members of the Nazi Party in 1935, only 5.5% were women; women were explicitly barred from top positions in the Nazi ranks as early as January, 1921, and Nazi medical philosophers were quite explicit about their feelings on this matter. A 1933 editorial of the journal of the Nazi Physicians' League announced that the National Socialist movement was "the most masculine movement to have appeared in centuries."

One of the initial thrusts of Nazi policy was to take women out of the workplace and return them to the home, where they were to have as many children as possible. Fritz Lenz, for example, argued that any woman with fewer than 15 babies (!) by menopause should be considered pathological. The government was more modest, pushing what it called the *four-child family* ideal. On December 16, 1938, Hitler announced the establishment of the Honor Cross of German Motherhood (modeled on the Iron Cross), awarded in bronze for four children, silver for six, and gold for eight.[10] After 1938, all public officials (including professors) were required to marry or else resign; medical journals published the names of unmarried or childless colleagues.

Nazi population policy, directed toward what Interior Minister Frick called "the solution to the woman question," was remarkably successful. The birth rate jumped from 14.7/

1000 in 1933 to 18/1000 in 1934, representing what Friedrich Burgdörfer called an unprecedented achievement in world population history, and a victory in the "war of births."

Yet, the German victory was one that set efforts at women's liberation back nearly 100 years. According to official Nazi policy, unmarried women were not considered citizens but were relegated instead to the status of *Staatsangehöriger* (deprived, that is, of certain rights), to which Jews were also initially assigned. As of 1936, women were banned from becoming lawyers, judges, and a host of other professions; quotas on the proportion of female students at German universities were reinstated.

At the same time that forced sterilization and abortion were instituted for individuals of inferior genetic stock, sterilization and abortion for "healthy" German women were declared illegal and punishable (in some cases by death) as a "crime against the German body." (Bavaria's official medical journal declared abortion a form of treason.) Access to birth control in all forms was also severely curtailed—except of course for Jews, for whom birth control was generally available and encouraged.

It is not well known, but there is one final aspect of gender that has escaped most discussions of the holocaust. In 1939, there were substantially more Jewish women in Germany than Jewish men; indeed, the ratio was roughly 14 women for every 10 men[11] (men had presumably managed to emigrate in greater numbers). Historians have largely ignored the fact that among German Jews killed in concentration camps (including most of the 167,000 Jews living in Germany in 1941), some 60% were women. Women also outnumbered men among the Gypsies killed at Auschwitz.[12]

The Nuremberg Laws

In the fall of 1935, Hitler signed into law the so-called Nuremberg Laws—excluding Jews from citizenship and preventing marriage or sexual relations between Jews and non-Jews. A further measure, the Marital Health Laws, required couples to submit to medical examination before marriage to see if "racial pollution" might be involved.

I cannot go into detail here on the operation of these laws; the story has been told elsewhere.[13] Let me simply point out that the Nuremberg Laws were considered public health measures and were administered primarily by physicians. In early 1936, when the Marital Health Laws went into effect, responsibility for administering the laws fell to marital counseling centers established in the Weimar period. The centers were greatly expanded beginning in 1935; they were renamed "genetic counseling centers" and attached to local public health offices. The Nuremberg Laws, along with the Sterilization Law, were two of the primary reasons expenditures and personnel for public health actually expanded under the Nazis.

I should also note that as with the Sterilization Law, here, too, German racial theorists learned from the Americans. In 1932, Bavarian Health Inspector Walter Schultze noted that the US must be regarded as a nation where "racial policy and thinking has become much more popular than in other countries." Schultze was referring not just to sterilization laws, but to American immigration restriction laws—especially the 1924 Immigration Restriction Act, the major consequence of which was to cut annual immigration into the US by about 95%.

In subsequent years, racial hygienists looked to other aspects of American racial policy for instruction. Nazi physicians on more than one occasion argued that German racial policies were relatively liberal compared with the way blacks were treated in the US. Evidence for this was usually taken from the fact that in several southern states, a person with 1/32 black ancestry was legally black, whereas if someone was 1/8 Jewish in Germany (and for many purposes, 1/4 Jewish), that person was legally Aryan. Nazi physicians spent a great deal of time discussing American miscegenation legislation; German medical journals reproduced charts showing the states in which blacks could or could not marry whites, could or could not vote, and so forth.

In 1939, Germany's leading racial hygiene journal reported that the University of Missouri had refused to admit black students. The same year, the journal reported the recent refusal of the American Medical Association to admit black physicians to its membership. German physicians had only recently (in 1938) barred Jews from practicing medicine (except on other Jews); racial theorists were thereby able to argue that Germany was not alone in its efforts to preserve racial purity.[14]

Euthanasia

In early October 1939, Hitler issued orders that certain doctors be commissioned to grant "a mercy death" (*Gnadentod*) to patients judged "incurably sick by medical examination." By August 1941, when the so-called "euthanasia" operation was largely brought to a close (*see below*,), more than 70,000 patients from German mental hospitals had been killed in an operation that provided the stage rehearsal for the subsequent destruction of Jews, homosexuals, Communists, Gypsies, Slavs, and prisoners of war.

The idea of the destruction of "lives not worth living" did not begin with the Nazis but had been discussed in legal and medical literature long before the Nazi rise to power. And not just in Germany. In 1935, the same year Egas Moniz invented the lobotomy, the French-American Nobel Prize winner Alexis Carrel suggested in his book *Man the Unknown* that the criminal and mentally ill should be "humanely and economically disposed of in small euthanasia institutions supplied with proper gases." Six years later, as German psychiatrists were sending the last of their patients into the gas chambers, an article appeared in the *Journal of the American Psychiatric Association* calling for the killing of retarded children, "nature's mistakes."[15]

The fundamental argument for forcible euthanasia was economic; euthanasia was justified as a kind of preemptive triage to free up beds. This became especially important in war time. I want to stress this: Things can happen in war that would not be tolerated in peacetime. And in fact, the euthanasia operation was consciously timed to coincide with the invasion of Poland. The first gassings of mental patients occurred at Posen, in Poland, on October 15, 1939, just 45 days after the invasion of that country marked the beginning of World War II.[16] In Germany itself, after the end of the first phase of the killing in August 1941, euthanasia became part of normal hospital routine. Handicapped infants were regularly put to death; persons requiring long-term psychiatric care and judged "incurable" suffered a similar fate. The war economy claimed many victims: After bombing attacks made space short, psychiatric institutes were cleared out (their patients murdered) to make up for lost space. In at least one instance, a home for the elderly was emptied in this fashion—its inhabitants sent to Meseritz-Obrawalde in Poland, where they were killed.[17]

The importance of war can also be seen in the fact that during World War I, half of all German mental patients starved to death, 45,000 in Prussia alone according to one estimate. They were simply too low on the list to receive rations. In the Nazi period, starvation of the mentally ill, the homeless, and other "useless eaters" became official state policy after a prolonged propaganda campaign to stigmatize the mentally ill and handicapped as "lives not worth living."

One should recall that the euthanasia program was planned and administered by leading figures in the German medical community. When the first experiments to test gasses for killings took place in Brandenburg Hospital in January 1940, Viktor Brack, head of the operation, emphasized that such gassings "should be carried out only by physicians." Brack cited the motto, *The needle belongs in the hand of the doctor.*

It is also important to appreciate the banality and the popularity of the euthanasia operation. In 1941, for example, the psychiatric hospital at Hadamar celebrated the cremation of its 10,000th patient in a special ceremony, where everyone in attendance—secretaries, nurses, and psychiatrists—received a bottle of beer for the occasion. The operation was also popular outside the medical community. Parents were made to feel shame and embarrassment at having to raise an abnormal or malformed child. Hospital archives are filled with letters from parents writing to health authorities requesting their children be granted euthanasia.

Historians exploring the origins of the Nazi destruction of "lives not worth living" have only in recent years begun to stress the link between the euthanasia operation on the one hand and the Final Solution on the other. And yet, the two programs were linked in both theory and practice. The most important theoretical link was what might be called the "medicalization of antisemitism," part of a broader effort to reduce a host of social problems—unemployment, homosexuality, crime, antisocial behavior, and so on—to medical or ideally surgical problems.

The "Jewish question," for example, was commonly cast as a public health problem. One of the leading research priorities in this period was to study the racial specificity of disease (I mentioned earlier the case of blood-group research). In 1935, when Gerhard Wagner addressed the Nuremberg Party Congress, he was able to cite extensive medical research proving that various "diseases," including homosexuality, insanity, feeble-mindedness, hysteria, suicide, gallstones, bladder and kidney stones, neuralgia, chronic rheumatism, and flat feet, were more common among Jews than non-Jews. In the same speech in which he proposed destruction of the mentally ill, Wagner declared that "Judaism is disease incarnate."

The medicalization of deviance continued into the war years. The first Nazi-administered Jewish ghettoes in Poland, for example, were justified in terms of a quarantine; permission to enter or leave the ghettoes was granted only by medical authorities. This, of course, eventually also became a self-fulfilling prophecy. Medical journals in the early 1940s denounced Jews as a diseased race and were able to invoke statistics on typhus levels in the Warsaw ghetto to prove the point.[18]

In the course of the late 1930s, German scientists proposed a number of different solutions to the Jewish question. The agronomist Hans Hefelmann suggested exporting all Jews to Madagascar. Dr. Philip Bouhler proposed sterilizing all Jews by X-rays. Viktor Brack recommended sterilization of the 2–3 million Jews capable of work, who might be put to use in Germany's factories. German medical authorities also devoted themselves to this problem: During the early war years the official journal of the German Medical Association, *Deutsches Aerzteblatt*, published a regular column on "Solving the Jewish Question."

The ultimate decision to gas the Jews emerged from the fact that the technical apparatus already existed for the destruction of the mentally ill. In the fall of 1941, with the completion of the bulk of the euthanasia operation, the gas chambers at psychiatric hospitals were dismantled and shipped East, where they were reinstalled at Majdanek, Auschwitz, and Treblinka. The same doctors, technicians, and nurses often followed the equipment. In this sense, there were both theoretical and practical continuities between the destruction of the "lives not worth living" in Germany's mental hospitals and the destruction of Germany's ethnic and social minorities.

Conclusion

Most leading German physicians supported the Nazis. Why? Physicians commonly boasted that their profession had shown its allegiance earlier and in greater strength than any other professional group. But why?

First of all, we should recall that the medical profession at this time was quite conservative. Prior to 1933, the leadership of the profession was dominated by the *Deutschnationalen*, a German nationalist party that subsequently threw its sup-

port to Hitler. Not all physicians, of course, were conservative. The profession was politicized and polarized after the
economic collapse in the late 1920s and early 1930s; physicians moved from the center to the left or the right. The socialists (and communists), however, were always a minority
in the German medical community. By the end of 1932, the
Nazi Physicians' League was twice as large as the Association of Socialist Physicians (3,000 vs 1,500 members). In the
Reichstag elections leading to the Nazi seizure of power, nine
physicians were elected to represent the Nazi Party; only one
was elected to represent the socialists.

Apart from this conservatism, it is possible to argue that
there was a certain ideological affinity between medicine and
Nazism at this time. Many physicians were attracted by the
importance given to race in the Nazi view of the world. Race
at this time was generally considered a medical or anthropo-
logical concept (most anthropologists were trained as physicians); physicians were intrigued by the Nazi effort to
biologize or medicalize a broad range of social problems,
including crime, homosexuality, the falling birth rate, the collapse of German imperial strength, and the "Jewish and
Gypsy problems."

The Nazis, in turn, were able to exploit both the inti-
macy and the authority of the traditional physician–patient
relationship. Crudely put, you could do things with doctors
that would have been much harder without. Doctors served
as executioners on German submarines; they routinely performed "selections" (of people to be killed) in concentration
camps. Himmler recognized the special role of physicians in
this regard: on March 9, 1943, the Reichsführer of the SS
issued an order that henceforth, only physicians trained in
anthropology could perform selections at concentration
camps.[19] Medicine also served as a disguise. In Buchenwald,
7,000 Russian prisoners of war were executed in the course
of supposed medical exams, using a device disguised as an
instrument to measure height.

There is a further element. The rise of the Nazis coincides with a period of concern about what was widely known as the "crisis" in modern science and in medicine, a crisis associated with the increasing specialization and bureaucratization of science and traced alternatively to urbanization, capitalism, Bolshevism, materialism, or any of a host of other real and/or apparent threats to human health and well-being. The Nazis promised to restore Germany to a more natural (*biologische*) way of living. Nazi philosophers rejected separate sciences "for the laboratory and the bedside"; science in the new state would challenge Galileo's claim "to measure what is measurable, and make measurable what is not." Nazi philosophers promised a future with "more Goethe, and less Newton."

In such a climate, Jews became a convenient scapegoat for all that was wrong in modern medicine. This was especially easy because Jews were in fact quite prominent in the German medical profession: 60% of Berlin's physicians, for example, were either Jewish or of Jewish ancestry. Jews were blamed for the bureaucratization and scientization of medicine and were accused of transforming medicine from a calling into a trade, from an art into a business. National socialism promised to eliminate Jews from the profession, restoring the honor and status of the doctor.

And in a certain sense, the medical profession might even be said to have prospered under the Nazis. In terms of personnel and funding, the German medical community was enlarged under the Nazis despite the banishing of Jews and communists. It may even be true that physicians achieved a higher status in the Nazi period than at any time before or since. During the 12 years of Nazi rule, for example, the office of *Rektor* (president) at German universities was occupied by physicians about half of the time; this contrasts with 19% for the decade prior to the rise of the Nazis and 18% for the two decades following the Nazi period. Doctors also prospered financially under the Nazis. In 1926, lawyers earned an average annual salary of 18,000 RM, compared with only 12,000 RM for physicians. But by 1936, doctors had reversed this and now earned 2,000 RM more than lawyers.

The Nazis were, it is true, hostile to certain forms of theoretical science, especially certain forms of physics and mathematics. But they did support many areas of the sciences, especially the applied and engineering sciences and social sciences such as psychology and anthropology.[20] In the case of medicine, it is interesting that there is no massive exodus from the editorial boards of medical journals in the period 1932–1935. Medical journals did not close their doors. If you go to the New York Academy of Medicine, Stanford's Lane Library, or any other major medical library, you can find more than 150 German medical journals published continuously through the Nazi period—more than 100 meters of shelf space of journals! Few medical journals ceased publication in the early years of the regime; most of those that did cease publication did not close until the mid-war years.[21] In fact, some 30 odd new medical journals begin publishing during the Nazi period. Several of these are still published today.

Biomedical science was not, in other words, simply destroyed by the Nazis. The story is more complex. The Nazis suppressed some areas and encouraged others. The Nazis supported extensive research into ecology, public health, carcinogenesis, human genetics, criminal biology, and of course, racial hygiene and sociobiology.[22] The Nazi government funded elaborate research on the effects of exposure to X-rays and heavy metals; some of the first reliable studies of the health effects of asbestos were done in this period. The Nazis were the first (so far as I'm aware) to initiate bans on smoking in public buildings;[23] Nazi leaders organized massive support for midwifery, homeopathy, and a number of other areas of heterodox medicine. Nazi physicians recognized the importance of a diet high in fruit and fiber; the Nazis passed a law requiring every German bakery to produce whole-grain bread. Nazi physicians restricted the use of DDT, and denied women tobacco rationing coupons on the grounds that nicotine could harm the fetus. Nazi physicians stressed the importance of preventive rather than curative medicine; racial hygiene was supposed to provide long-run, preventive care for the German germ plasm, complementing shorter-term social and individual hygiene.

I have stressed the continuity with pre-1933 traditions; I do not have space here to discuss the important postwar continuities. Let me simply note in conclusion four points. First, it is important to appreciate not just the extent to which the Nazis were able to draw upon the imagery and authority of science but also the extent to which Nazi ideology informed the practice of science. Second, scientists were not bystanders or even pawns. Many (not all, but not a few) helped to construct the racial policies of the Nazi state. It is probably as fair to say that Nazi racial policy emerged from within the scientific community, as to say that it was imposed upon that community.

Third, it is commonly said that the Nazis politicized science and that much of what went wrong under the Nazis can be traced to this politicization. The argument I've made here is that one cannot consider the experience of the medical profession in terms of a simple use-and-abuse model of science. Among physicians, there were as many volunteers as victims: No one had to force physicians to support the regime. Hefelmann testified to this effect in the euthanasia trial at Limburg in 1964: "No doctor was ever ordered to participate in the euthanasia program; they came of their own volition."[24]

The Nazis did not have to politicize science; in fact, it is probably fair to say that the Nazis *depoliticized* science in the sense that they removed from science the political diversity that makes the politics of science (or medicine, or technology) interesting. The Nazis destroyed a vigorous socialist medical tradition that had transformed Weimar medical practice, establishing local outpatient clinics, self-help networks, and the like. The Nazis denounced the "political" as a category of discussion: The German state was to be a *Volksstaat*, not a *Parteistaat*; National Socialism was to be counted a movement, not a party. The Nazis sought to transform prob-

lems of racial, sexual, or social deviance into medical problems; Germany's social and political problems would be
solved by diagnosis, disinfection, and surgery. Murder was
practiced in the name of quarantine, apartheid in the name
of public health.

Finally, I do not want to leave the impression that the
horrors of this period can be attributed to anything inherent
in science or medicine, or even to technocracy or the rule of
technical elites. It took a powerful state to concentrate and
unleash the destructive forces within German medicine, and
without that state, science would have remained impotent
in this sphere. In the midst of a war engineered by an aggres-
sive, expansionistic state, Nazi ideologues were able to turn
to doctors and scientists to carry out programs that even
today stand as unexcelled exemplars of evil. The collaboration of scientists made this disturbingly easy, frightfully free
of hitches. Where was the resistance, and why was it so
feeble? Why were so many so willing to serve? The myth of
"following orders," invented for postwar tribunals, has never
been convincing. The questions remain.

From: *When Medicine Went Mad* Ed.: A. Caplan
©1992 The Humana Press Inc.

Eugenics

The Science and Religion of the Nazis

Benno Müller-Hill

Introduction

It was a mixture, or better, an amalgam of science, politics, and *Weltanschauung* (ideology or religion) that culminated in the project of the final solution of the Jewish question, or the Holocaust. Let me first define science: Science describes the world as it is. Proper science does not say what the world should look like. Something other than science—religion, ethics, conscience, or ideology—guides men and women on how to act in a society. Some scientists will not agree with this statement that essentially echoes Max Weber. I can see their reason. They spend all of their time in the laboratory or behind their desks. They have little to do with nonscientists. Their main—if not only—interest is science. Science tells them not only how their research object, usually a tiny part of the world, looks like, but also what they should do to understand it by manipulating it in the best possible manner. The experiments should be fast, elegant, and cheap. And if this is so in the laboratory, why not in society and the rest of the world? Is not society and the world a kind of laboratory in which all acts should be justified only scientifically? I think this view is more than a mistake; it is

43

fundamentally wrong. Sure, scientists create constructs and situations that demand decisions. They can point out risks and costs. They may favor a view where everything is decided only to minimize risks and costs, but that in itself is an ideology or religion.

Human Genetics and Eugenics, 1900–1933

Fifty years ago a human geneticist knew that the genotype of humans largely determines their phenotype and that differences in phenotype indicate differences in genotype. He believed that the mode of human thinking and feeling is determined to a large extent by the genotype. He noticed different behavior in humans and concluded that different genotypes may be the reason. Then, most human geneticists were fairly sure that the human genotype (nature) was much more influential than education, i.e., nurture. It should be noted that the term "human geneticist" may be misleading. At that time, DNA was not known to house the genes. Molecular biology did not exist. Only pedigrees could be studied, and no particular scientific training was needed to collect and analyze a human pedigree. Thus, psychologists and psychiatrists became human geneticists just by their ability to define human behavioral phenotypes.

It seemed then self-evident for the psychologists and psychiatrists to attribute values to the different human phenotypes. Healthy, sane, and intelligent were "good" phenotypes. Sick, insane, and mentally retarded were "bad" phenotypes. Language helped: In Germany, the chronically ill were routinely called "inferior" (*minderwertig*) and the healthy "superior" (*höherwertig*) by the medical profession. The Nazis echoed Nietzsche, when they talked about the *Übermensch* and the *Untermensch*. They all believed in the reality of the language they spoke.

Since the single psychiatric patient could not be helped by any treatment, it seemed almost obvious to disregard his plight and to concentrate on the problems all these patients caused to society. "The individual is almost nothing and society is everything," wrote Konrad Lorenz.[1] The Nazis simply omitted the "almost." Would it not be better for society that such "inferior" persons not be born or at least would not propagate? Moreover, the analysis of human populations in Europe and the US seemed to show that the "inferior" bred faster then the "superior." The eugenicists were deeply worried by this prospect. Western culture and civilization seemed seriously endangered. As responsible scientists, they felt something had to be done: They made various proposals. Negative measures (such as sterilizations or marriage laws) might stop propagation of the unwanted "inferior," and positive measures (such as tax laws) might encourage propagation of the "superior."

The human geneticists believed that such differences between inferior and superior phenotypes were to be found within any human race (i.e., a population with similar physical phenotypes). But they assumed too, that deep differences existed between various races. All of them believed Blacks were inferior in intelligence to Caucasians. But even when a particular race, such as the Jewish race, was not regarded as inferior, many human geneticists assumed that race mixing would bring negative effects. Therefore, most of them advocated measures against racial mixings.

Nowhere in Europe did the eugenicists have the strong goverment support they needed to make their vision reality. When the International Congress of Eugenics was held in Rome in 1929, the eugenicists approached Mussolini, imploring the dictator to adopt their program. But Mussolini was not interested. At the same time, it was impossible to pass a law in Germany that would allow the sterilization of persons against their will. The democratic parties were all against it. But it seemed possible to pass a law that would allow the sterilization of consenting patients. Consent of the feeble-minded and insane was, in this respect, consent of the persons representing their legal interest. This was thought by the eugenicists to be just a beginning. Such a law was in preparation before the Nazis came to power. The Nazis alone favored a law that would allow the sterilization of persons against their will or the will of the persons representing them. Such a hard law was thought by the eugenicists to be a prerequisite for all effective eugenic action.

Eugenics in Nazi Germany

The Nazis were of course known for their violent antisemitism and their antidemocratic goals. In spite of this, the leading non-Jewish German geneticists (Erwin Baur, Eugen Fischer, Fritz Lenz, Theodor Mollison, Ernst Rüdin) accepted the Nazis as partners before they came to power in order to get the desired eugenic legislation. These professors were no friends of democracy. They were all antisemitic to some extent. To differentiate themselves from their Jewish German colleagues active in eugenics, they preferred the term race hygiene to eugenics. For the Nazi politicians, this professorial antisemitism was much too weak. But since experts and Nazis needed each other, they accepted each other. The Nazis soon made the professors accept a much more violent antisemitism than they had confessed before. The Nazis gained the propagandistic and technical help to execute all their racial programs, and the experts got research money and the feeling of importance.

The Nazis tried to create a coherent Weltanschauung or religion for the proper use of the results of human genetics. This view was sufficiently coherent that one may call it a religion. It had its own sacred language. The believers did not speak of genes; they prayed to the blood. The word gene was the vernacular the scientists used, the word blood the sacred word for the believers. Only the crazy Nazi-fundamentalist (every religion has its fundamentalists) believed literally in the inheritance through blood. Those who differentiated correctly between science and religion but who accepted the Nazi religion were the real architects of Nazi Germany. This amalgam of science and Nazi ideology (or better, religion) produced the measures that culminated in the project of the murder of all Jews, the final solution of the

Jewish question, as they called it. I will now list some of these measures.[2,3] The list is incomplete. Outside of the scope of this article is particularly the merciless persecution of all those who politically opposed the Nazis, first communists and social democrats but later, also conservatives.

1933: Passing of a law that allowed compulsory sterilization of schizophrenics, the feeble-minded, and others. Between 1934 and 1939, about 350,000 persons were sterilized under this law.

1935: Passing of the Nuremberg law interdicting marriage and sexual contacts between Jews and other Germans.

1937: Illegal sterilization of a few hundred colored children and the start of a program to sterilize most of the 30,000 German Gypsies as part of an estimated 1 million of those unfit for modern German society. Most German Gypsies were murdered between 1943 and 1944 in Auschwitz.

1940: The illegal killing of about 70,000 German psychiatric patients by gas begins. It ends in summer, 1941. More than 100,000 patients die in the following years from hunger and infections. The psychiatric wards are as bad as the camps.

1941: Plans to sterilize all one-quarter Jews and to kill all full and half Jews. The mass murder of the Jews begins. The conditions in the camps and the psychiatric wards lead to the breakdown of all former ethics of medical research.

The destructive drive of Nazi ideology (religion) invaded the realm of science proper. Secrecy invited lying, and lack of discussion invited fraud. Many experimenters got carried away and forgot normal scientific practice. The anatomist Professor August Hirt, the psychiatrist Professor Carl Schneider, and the gynecologist Professor Carl Clauberg are examples of this process. Yet these medical scientists remained respected members of the German scientific establishment right up to their suicidal ends. It should be kept in mind that some of the scientific work done was first class, the neuroanatomical work of Professor Julius Hallervorden for example.

Medical scientists were involved in all the programs mentioned above. The statement that the various human populations were genetically significantly different was presumably correct, but the value statement that one race (population) was *superior* to the other was unscientific and pure ideology and religion. Thus human genetics and eugenics in Germany turned into a religion and a religious cult. This amalgam between eugenics and antisemitism was particularly destructive. It is most significant in this context that the Jews and the Gypsies and the chronically insane (the schizophrenics) were degraded to occupy the lowest rank in Nazi Europe. Those who thought differently, allegedly forced by their genes, had to disappear. They were deprived of all human rights and were worked to death or killed directly.

The Nazis thought the disappearance of the insane would guarantee a sane world; the disappearance of the Gypsies together with all those unfit for modern society would guarantee a productive world without petty crime. They thought the disappearence of the Jews would help economic planning of conquered Europe and would guarantee a world free from Jewish thinking. The orthodox Jews particularly lived their lives in total opposition to these Nazi values. According to the Torah, the insane should be cared for and not killed. Every single life should be regarded as worthy as any other. The Gentiles should be treated as justly as the fellow Jews and not robbed of their rights. God and not blood or destiny should be praised. The Jewish religion was indeed the absolute opposite of the Nazi religion. So, it had to be destroyed with its believers if the Nazi religion was to win.

Discussion

Ethical Implications

The message from Auschwitz is different for different people. But a common ground for Jews and nonJews may be found in the following considerations: The attempt of science to provide acceptable values and ethics has failed. Medicine and science should never again be trusted when they promise to deliver their own ethical values; these values have to come from other sources. The destruction of German synagogues and the annihilation of Jewish believers and nonbelievers alike should have a deep impact on the thinking of non-Jews to rediscover the Pentateuch and essential Jewish thinking. Whatever is found to be against it should be permanently questioned and possibly abandoned.

Data Obtained Criminally Should Not Be Used

The question has been often raised whether data from Nazi experiments should be used if potentially they might save human lives. I would like to discuss here two extreme cases. The first deals with Huntington's chorea. Patients having this disease had to be sterilized according to the German sterilization law of 1933. But the first signs of real illness appear only when the patient is about 40 years old. In general, he is then already a parent. It was thus suggested by German psychiatrists that persons from families with Huntington's chorea should be sterilized as young as possible if they showed any sign of possible psychic anomalies announcing a possible later outbreak of the disease. A dissertation[4] suggests that about 1% of those sterilized from 1934 to 1940 were patients with suspected Huntington's chorea. This would amount to approximately 3,500 persons sterilized for that reason. Records of these family studies survived the war. Should these records be used today to spot families with carriers of Huntington's chorea? I think definitely not; too much injustice has been done to these families. If they like to see a medical doctor they are free to do that, but they should not be approached by geneticists or doctors interested in the disease. Yet, this has been done by Dr. Herwig Lange from Düsseldorf Medical School.

On the other end of the spectrum are the Rascher experiments. They have been discussed extensively in the media and also at a recent conference on bioethics.[5] There, a medical scientist (Dr. Robert Pozos), two bioethicists (Drs. Benjamin Freedman and Velvl Greene), and one historian of

science (Dr. Robert Proctor) agreed that Rascher's cooling
data should be used to save human lives. I contradict this
opinion and would like to outline my specific arguments. The
history of Dr. Sigmund Rascher has been described in a book[6]
and an article.[7] I argue on two levels: The first level is purely
scientific, the second is nonscientific and what some may call
religious. I come again to only one conclusion: The data should
be taboo. We should remember those who died. We should
not try to squeeze a profit out of it.

Rascher was a fraud. The files of the *Deutsche
Forschungsgemeinschaft* (DFG) indicate that the work he did
in 1936–1938 while getting a stipend from the DFG was a
fake. He described a spectacular test for cancer that could
not be reproduced. Under normal circumstances, such a person is barred from further research, and if he manages to go
on with research, his data would be looked upon with
extreme suspicion. Rascher indeed could not advance his
medical career within normal channels. He approached
Himmler, a friend of his wife, and got the position of a
researcher at Dachau concentration camp. Work he did there
was again spurious. Together with a known fraudulent
researcher, Dr. Karl Fahrenkamp, Rascher published a paper
on a revolutionary drug against bleeding and for wound-heal-
ing. The concoction, "polygal," was without any value, but
several persons were severely wounded by Rascher's gun-
shots. Finally, the techniques of recording the process of
dying in cold water were those of 40 years ago. I presume
they were inaccurate, never mind the urge of cheating that
drove Rascher. By their very nature, these murders cannot
be reproduced. In summary, they lack all ingredients of trustworthy scientific data. I thought no proper scientist would
touch them. I was wrong, Dr. Pozos did.[5]

I may add here that Rascher was a fraud in his private
life, too. His wife did not get the children Himmler expected
her to have. So she faked pregnancies and somehow bought
three children. She stole the fourth from a woman at the
Munich train station. The police caught her. Her husband
was called as a witness by the police. He claimed to know

nothing and appealed to Himmler, but Himmler had them both jailed and finally executed.

Now, let us assume that the data had been properly recorded and reproduced. I think there is still good reason not to use such data. To argue that saving human lives would finally give back dignity and value to the murdered and thereby give sense to the murders is outrageous: It honors the murderer and not the murdered. I would have hoped that anyone who thought it was the other way around would have been shattered in his convictions after reading accounts of witnesses from Auschwitz, such as those of Mrs. Mozes-Kor and Mrs. Seiler-Vigorito in this volume. I thought a stone would be moved hearing their arguments against the use of such data. But in spite of that, a majority of ethicists is apparently in favor of their use.[5] I even heard the argument that the emotions gained by their experience in Auschwitz disqualified the victims from judging the issue. It seems to me that this amounts to the idolatry of science. Religious Jews know that idolatry should not be committed. They know that idolatry, murder, and adultery are the three things you should not do to save your own life. I have tried to show here and elsewhere that genetics and eugenics turned into the religion of the Nazis. The religion of the Nazis was a Baal's religion where millions were sacrificed on the altars, the ovens they erected in Auschwitz and elsewhere.

Scientists must learn that truth is not the supreme value. Science should be a servant not the master of humankind. Kant argued that you have to tell a killer the road to his victim, if he asks you:[8] Truth has to be honored always, according to this German philosopher. German geneticists thought that Jewish paternity determinations were a purely scientific problem, even as late as 1943. It was not their problem that the persons they declared Jewish lost their civil rights and had to travel first to Theresienstadt and later to Auschwitz. As geneticists, they did science only. The view that science alone determines what has to be done is idolatry. It has to be resisted, or we are spiritually back in the late 1920s before the beginning of Nazi Germany.

The Human Genome Proiect

The consideration of Nazi eugenics and Rascher's data is not only a matter of history. They are particularly relevant for the future of the Human Genome Project. Through this project, some differences in human phenotypes will be scientifically proven to be owing to different genotypes. Some of these genotypes will correctly be seen as the cause of disablement or nonfunction of their carriers in the industrial society of the 21st century. What will have prevalence? Scientific truth or the dignity of the afflicted person? Will the bioethicists who approved the use of Rascher's data approve of the idea that employers, insurance companies, or just anyone will have the right to ask a person about his genotype? Will they agree that employers or insurance companies have the right to deny employment or insurance to those who refuse to have their genotype revealed? Will they condone the notion that a woman should be punished because she has an abortion for reasons they do not approve of and punished again when she refuses to have an abortion when they forecast high costs and no return? Will they argue again that human lives have to be saved with dubious data? Their willingness to use Rascher's data lead me to expect the worst.

I have until now believed that this could never happen, precisely because the Holocaust happened. I am beginning to realize that I may have been wrong. Sometimes at night, I see the faces of the two German eugenicists Eugen Fischer and Erwin Rüdin smile. I hear them mumble to each other that now they may be vindicated as the forerunners who made the inevitable mistakes of scientific progress. And I hear them laugh. What wonderful times ahead of them.

It is not yet too late. Let me repeat: No person should have the right to inquire as to the genotype of any other person. Any such attempt by an employer or an insurance company should be punishable by law. There is still time to act.

From: *When Medicine Went Mad* Ed.: A. Caplan
©1992 The Humana Press Inc.

How Did Medicine Go So Wrong?

Arthur L. Caplan

Is Moral Inquiry
into Nazi Medical Crimes Immoral?

Analysis of the ethical issues raised by "experimentation" or medical "treatments" carried out by German physicians and scientists during the time of the Third Reich must be approached with great caution. Talk of ethics seems, at the least, incongruous when the conduct being discussed involves the mass murder of innocent persons. Even to talk of ethics is to risk conferring legitimacy on the patently illegitimate.

The myriad crimes carried out under medical supervision in Germany prior to and during World War II were so heartless, cruel, and inhumane that it is not at all evident why it is necessary to subject them to moral analysis. Is there any reason to conduct an ethical analysis of Nazi medical crimes? The conduct of German biomedicine during the Nazi era was *prima facie* abhorrent and indisputably immoral. There is no need for an argument to prove that what happened was evil.

Despite the obvious immorality of biomedicine's role in the Holocaust, there is, nevertheless, a need for moral inquiry; it is necessary to understand how those who committed horrific crimes on a massive scale were able to persuade themselves that what they were doing was ethically correct. As difficult as it is to accept, some physicians, public health officials, nurses, and government agencies killed, maimed, tortured, or did not protest these activities because they believed it was morally correct to perform them.

Still, treating in a serious manner the ethical arguments made by a scientist to justify the acquisition of physiological information by slowly freezing dozens of men to death strains the boundaries of moral discourse. Taking seriously the moral rationales made by a doctor for using massive doses of radiation to surreptitiously sterilize a 12-year-old girl risks both trivializing ethical analysis and permitting exculpation for the foulest of deeds.

There is another danger involved in subjecting the moral arguments of Nazi health care professionals to ethical analysis. Evaluating the moral defense offered by those in German medicine and science who participated actively in the Holocaust in the same tone, discourse, and style that is used to mull over the fine points of informed consent or physician-patient confidentiality in contemporary German, British, or American medicine suggests a moral equivalence between the deeds and the times. Using the same analytical tools to look at mass murder and the protection of medical confidentiality may lead some to conclude that the offenses of the past were no worse than the problems that arise today in the practice of medicine.[1]

The inadvertent transformation of evil by the attempt to understand the rationales offered for it is a very real risk of subjecting Nazi medical crimes to analysis, moral or otherwise.[2] But transformation, exculpation, and trivialization need not be necessary consequences of raising ethical questions about what doctors and scientists said in defense of their conduct in the camps, mental asylums, and nursing homes of the Third Reich.

The horrors, crimes, and abuses of biomedicine in the Third Reich were staggering in their scope. Millions of people, people innocent of any crime or wrongdoing, people who had neither arms nor, for many, the ability to wage armed struggle against the Third Reich were tortured, mutilated, starved, and murdered as threats to the state. Babies were killed only because of their race, religion, or mental physical disability. There can be no doubt that these acts were immoral and evil. But those who carried out mass murder, sterilization, and cruel experiments did so for reasons they believed were moral. This fact is difficult to accept for those who take ethics seriously. However, by avoiding a confrontation with the ethical justifications provided by biomedicine for its role in the Holocaust, a number of dangerous and distorting myths about that role are able to flourish.

Debunking the Myths
of Incompetence, Madness, and Coercion

It is comforting to believe that health care professionals who have pledged an oath to "do no harm" and who are minimally concerned with the morality of their own conduct could not kill babies or conduct brutal, often lethal, experiments on starving inmates in concentration camps. It is comforting to think that it is not possible to defend involuntary euthanasia, forced sterilization, and genocide in moral terms. It is comforting to think that anyone who espouses racist, eugenic ideas cannot be a competent, introspective physician or scientist. Such beliefs are especially comforting to ethicists. Nazi medical crimes show that each of these beliefs is false.

It is commonly believed that only madmen, charlatans, and incompetents among doctors, scientists, public health officials, and nurses could possibly have associated with those who ran the Nazi party. Among those who did their *research* in Auschwitz, Dachau, and other camps, a considerable number had obvious psychological problems, were lesser scientific lights, or both.[2,3] But there were also well-trained, reputable, and competent physicians and scientists who were ardent Nazis. Some conducted experiments in the camps. Others decided who ought be put to death. Human experimentation in the camps was not conducted only by those who were mentally unstable or on the periphery of science. Support for genocide was not confined to the fringe of German medicine and science. Not all who engaged in experimentation or murder were inept (*see* Proctor, this volume and Müller-Hill, this volume).

Placing all of the physicians, health professionals, and scientists who took part in the crimes of the Holocaust on the periphery of medicine and science allows another myth to flourish—that medicine and science went mad when Adolf Hitler took control of Germany. Those physicians and public health officials who staffed the camps, murdered the demented, and advanced theories of racial hygiene were, according to this myth, simply lunatics, charlatans, and quacks. The myth of madness disguises all those who carried out crimes in the camps as incorrigible fiends, such as Josef Mengele,[2,4] or suffering from pathological personality disorders, such as Sigmund Rascher (*see* Berger, this volume). Competent and responsible physicians and scientists could not willingly have had anything to do with such evil deeds. However, the actions as well as the beliefs of German physicians and scientists under Nazism stand in glaring contrast to this myth.[5,6]

Once identified, the myths of incompetency and madness make absolutely no sense. How could flakes, crackpots, and incompetents have been the only ones supporting Nazism? Could the Nazis have had any chance of carrying out genocide on a staggering, monumental scale against victims scattered over half the globe without the zealous help of competent biomedical and scientific authorities? The technical and logistical problems of collecting, transporting, exploiting, murdering, scavenging, and disposing of the bodies of millions from dozens of nations required competence and skill, not ineptitude and madness.

The Holocaust differs from other instances of genocide in that it involved the active participation of medicine and science. The Nazis turned to biomedicine specifically for help in carrying out genocide after their early experience using specially trained troops to murder in Poland and the Soviet Union proved impractical (*see* Appendix).

Elite *SS* troops, specially trained in mass killing, found it psychologically impossible to, on a daily basis, use machine guns and pistols at point blank range to kill tens of thousands of persons and dump their bodies into mass graves. The psychological toll of this mode of genocide on the killers was too great. A solution was needed if genocide was to continue at a rapid pace on a mass scale.

The German biomedical and scientific communities provided the solution in the forms of medically supervised death camps. These camps were designed to permit effective, efficient means of impersonal killing. Poison gas, used in conjunction with crematoria, permitted mass killing with minimal contact between those who died and those who killed. It would not have been possible to achieve genocide on the desired scale and at the desired pace without the willing assistance of competent technological and biomedical expertise.

Another myth that has flourished in the absence of a serious analysis of the moral rationales proffered by those in biomedicine who participated in the Holocaust is that those who participated were coerced. Many doctors, nurses, and scientists in Germany and other nations have consoled themselves about the complicity of German medicine and science in genocide with the fable that once the Nazi regime seized power, the cooperation of the biomedical and scientific establishments was only secured by force.[2,5,6] Even then, this myth has it, cooperation among doctors, scientists, and public health officials with Nazism was grudging.

In recent years, it has become clear how intimate the association was between mainstream biomedical science and Nazism.[5,6,7] Mainstream biomedicine in Germany boarded the Nazi bandwagon early, stayed on for the duration of the Nazi regime, and suffered few public second thoughts or doubts about the association even after the collapse of the Reich.

The myths of incompetence, madness, and coercion have obscured the behavior of biomedicine under Nazism. This helps to explain the relative silence in the field of bioethics about both the conduct and justifications of those in biomedicine who were so intimately involved with the Nazi state.

Why Does Bioethics Have so Little To Say
About the Holocaust?

Among the various fields of scholarly inquiry, one that could reasonably be expected to have much to say about the role of biomedicine in the Holocaust is bioethics. Yet, scholars in bioethics have actually had relatively little to say about the Holocaust. If one dates the field of bioethics from the creation of the first bioethics institutes and university programs in the US in the mid-1960s, then the field is roughly 25 years old. Incredibly, no book-length bioethical study exists examining the actions, policies, abuses, crimes, or rationales of German doctors and biomedical scientists.

Anthologies and textbooks in the field of bioethics pay scant attention to the Nazi era. The most popular anthologies used in classrooms often have sections on the ethics of human experimentation but reprint only one or two articles about Nazi medical crimes or make no mention of the Holocaust at all.[8-11] Even review articles and books on the history of human experimentation and informed consent tend to devote relatively little space to discussing German medicine and science in the 1930s and 1940s. There is little evidence in the citations and footnotes of bioethics that those working in the field in the 1960s were greatly influenced by the Holocaust, the Nuremberg trials, or the promulgation of the Nuremberg Code to govern human experimentation.[12]

There has been almost no discussion of the roles played by medicine and science during the Nazi era in bioethics literature. Rather than see Nazi biomedicine as morally bad, the field of bioethics has generally accepted the myths that Nazi biomedicine was either inept, mad, or coerced. By subscribing to these myths, bioethics has been able to avoid a painful confrontation with the fact that many who committed the crimes of the Holocaust were competent physicians and health care professionals acting from their moral convictions. Not one of the doctors or public health officials on trial at Nuremberg pleaded for mercy on the grounds of insanity. A few claimed they were merely following legitimate orders, but no one alleged coercion.

The bitter reality is that the ranks of physicians, scientists, and public health officials who committed terrible acts against innocent persons included competent health professionals and scientists, some of international renown. Mainstream German medicine supported the rise of the Nazi party to power. Some of its leaders helped create the scientific foundation for the euthanasia program that was instituted to eliminate the disabled, demented, deformed, and, eventually, Jews and Gypsies. Others helped design the death camps. Most were neither mad nor coerced into cooperation with the Nazi regime. They believed what they were doing was right.

When called to account for their actions, Nazi doctors, scientists, and public health officials were surprisingly forthright about their reasons for their conduct. The same cannot be said for the ethical evaluations offered in Germany and in the West for their crimes. A fog of excuses, lies, and exculpation has been laid over the crematoria and laboratories of the concentration camps.[13] History has been rewritten to limit participation to the inept and the inapt. The biomedical community, both in Germany and in other nations, was not able to bring itself to admit that many of its peers—able physicians, doctors, nurses, public health officials, geneticists, and anthropologists in the most scientifically and technologically advanced society of its day—had supported and then flourished under a regime as vile as that of the Nazis.[7,14]

The puzzle of how it came to be that physicians and scientists who committed so many crimes and caused so much suffering and death did so in the belief that they were morally right cries out for analysis, discussion, and debate. But it is tremendously painful for those in bioethics to have to undertake such an analysis.

It if often presumed, if only tacitly, by those who teach bioethics that those who know what is ethical will not behave in immoral ways. What is the point of doing bioethics, of teaching courses on ethics to medical, nursing, and public health students, if the vilest and most horrendous of deeds and policies can be justified by moral reasons? Bioethics has been speechless in the face of the crimes of Nazi doctors and biomedical scientists precisely because so many of these doctors and scientists believed they were doing what was morally right to do.

The Nazi Analogy in Contemporary Bioethics

For all the lack of attention to the specific acts and rationales of German medicine during the Holocaust, there is no shortage of references to Nazism in contemporary debates about the ethics of medicine and science. Debates about abortion, the use of fetal tissue for medical purposes, euthanasia, and ongoing efforts to map and sequence the human genome are rife with warnings about and analogies to the Holocaust and to Nazism. The analogies take three major forms. The first uses the events of the Holocaust to illustrate where slippery slopes can lead. For example, critics of attempts to legalize both passive and active euthanasia often claim that permitting either will send us down the slope that Nazi physicians followed from killing the handicapped at Herborn to operating "showers" at Auschwitz.

The second type of analogy is used to show that something that is happening now is exactly analogous to what the Nazis did. Abortion is often referred to by those who would prohibit the practice as a modern day Holocaust (*see* Neuhaus, this volume). Killing millions of innocent Jews 50 years ago in camps in Poland is, according to some, morally the same as killing millions of innocent fetuses in abortion clinics in the US. Euthanasia also elicits this sort of analogy. Allowing a feeding tube to be withdrawn from a young woman in a permanent vegetative state in a Missouri nursing home in 1990 is the same conduct as allowing a handicapped infant to starve to death in a home for the feeble in Germany in 1939.

The third sort of analogy locates similarities between the rationales given for immoral conduct by Nazis and the attempts to defend what is seen as immoral conduct today.

For example, those who justify the use of fetal tissue for transplantation or research on the grounds that it is not wrong to take advantage of the availability of fetal remains to help others[15] are said to be echoing the rationales given by German scientists for their experiments on innocent concentration camp inmates.[16]

The absence of comment and discussion about exactly what Nazi biomedicine did and why allows these three types of analogies to proliferate unencumbered by facts. The only way to assess the validity of such analogies is to look closely at what German physicians and scientists did and the moral rationales they gave for their actions, in order to ascertain the extent of similarities between what happened then and what is happening now. In my opinion, many of the analogies and references made to the actions of Nazi doctors and scientists prior to and during the Holocaust are false and misleading, but this can only be shown if the actions and rationales of the Nazis are carefully analyzed.

To What Extent Was Biomedicine Involved with Nazism?

There are many ways in which complicity in an evil act or policy arises. Obviously, those who actively plan and carry out immoral acts are responsible for the evil that results. There can be no doubt that some physicians and scientists were complicit in this sense in perpetrating the horrors of the Holocaust.

Josef Mengele, a physician trained in human genetics, cruelly experimented upon and killed many young children whom he found of scientific interest because they were twins. He also selected for killing tens of thousands of men, women, and children at the gates of Auschwitz.[2,4] Gerhard Rose, head of the prestigious Koch Institute of Tropical Medicine, did conduct lethal experiments to develop a vaccine against typhus in a concentration camp. Many doctors killed those sent to camps or medical institutions by means of lethal injections or gassing.

Whereas it is known that some German physicians and scientists tortured and killed innocent persons, many histories of the Nazi era concentrate on the direct involvement in killing of a relatively small number of biomedical scientists and thus ignore or downplay the broad complicity of German medicine and science with Nazism. Ironically, even the postwar legal proceedings against war criminals tended to lend weight to the view that relatively few doctors or scientists killed, tortured, or murdered in the name of the Nazi state. Fewer than 100 physicians and only a handful of scientists and public health officials were found guilty by Allied courts and sentenced to prison or death for criminal acts. In order to win convictions for crimes for which there were few legal or judicial precedents, the prosecution had to emphasize those acts for which direct evidence of a clearcut crime existed.[17]

However, there are other ways in which moral responsibility and thus complicity can come to exist between individuals and immoral acts. People may bear responsibility for evil acts if they provide motives or rationales for others to undertake evil acts; or, they may be complicitous for their failure to protest or resist immoral actions or policies. It is easy, and for some tempting, to dismiss the acts of those who actually were tried and convicted at Nuremberg and other trials as the crazed behavior of an atypical, deviant minority who did not represent the mainstream of German medicine or science. Although widely accepted, the minimalization of the connection between biomedicine and Nazism does not square with reality.

Recent scholarship on the role played by medicine and biomedical sciences in fostering and supporting Nazi ideology and the Nazi state shows that far more than fringe elements of medicine and science were staunch supporters of the Nazi party and its programs.[1,2,5–7,14] Nor were these supporters dragged kicking, screaming, and protesting into involvement with the Nazi party and its actions. Physicians, nurses, public health officials, and biological and behavioral scientists in many cases did not have to be forced or coerced into participation in the formulation and support of systematic policies to exterminate Jews, Slavs, Gypsies, homosexuals, and other so-called inferior groups. The sequence of events that led to genocide, murder, torture, sterilization, and exploitation depended on the support and involvement of large segments of medicine, health care, and the sciences. Moreover, medicine and science were not particularly distinguished in their resistance to the Nazi party or its ideology.[2,6]

Whereas a relatively small number of doctors and scientists took an active and direct role in killing or torture, a large number, many in universities and prestigious institutes, provided intellectual, political, and professional support for the murderous policies of the Nazi state. Nazi ideology was firmly rooted in racial biology. The racism of Nazism was promulgated by internationally respected, mainstream German scientists and physicians who had numerous counterparts in the US, Great Britain, Canada, and other Western nations (see Proctor, this vol).[4,5,7,14] Euthanasia and genocide were couched in medical and public health terminology provided by prominent German physicians and public health officials. The technological challenge of transporting tens of millions of persons, selecting those suitable for slave labor, killing the rest, and then disposing of their remains required the active participation of German science, medicine, and engineering.

The Holocaust occurred with the intellectual support and involvement of the medical and scientific establishment of the most scientifically and technologically advanced society of its time. The Holocaust, unlike many other instances of mass killing, was scientifically inspired, supervised, and mediated genocide.

Those in medicine and the biological sciences were early and ardent supporters of Nazism and later of the Nazi state. The roots of Nazi racism found fertile soil in the race hygiene theories that dominated German medicine and biology before the ascendency of Hitler and the Nazi party to power. The ties between mainstream biomedicine and Nazism were so strong that many of those who supported the Nazi state and its actions retained their positions of authority and power long after the Nazi state had been defeated (see Appendix).

Experimentation in the Camps

Although the role of mainstream medicine and science in the Holocaust has been underplayed, there has been at least an acknowledgment that medicine and science perpetrated heinous crimes in the name of experimentation in the concentration camps. Yet, the scope of experimentation conducted in the camps is not widely understood.

There were at least 26 different types of experiments conducted for the explicit purpose of research in concentration camps or using concentration camp inmates in Germany, Poland, and France during the Nazi era. Among the studies in which human beings were used in research were the analysis of high-altitude decompression on the human body; attempts to make sea water drinkable; the efficacy of sulfanilamide for treating gunshot wounds; the feasibility of bone, muscle, and joint transplants; the ability to treat burns caused by incendiary bombs; the efficacy of polygal for treating trauma-related bleeding; the efficacy of high-dose radiation in causing sterility; the efficacy of phenol (gasoline) injections as a euthanasia agent; the efficacy of electroshock therapy; the symptoms and course of noma (starvation-caused skin gangrene); the postmortem examination of skeletons and brains to assess the effects of starvation; the efficacy of surgical techniques for sterilizing women; and the impact of stress and starvation on ovulation, menstruation, and cancerous growths in the reproductive organs of women. A variety of other studies were carried out on twins, dwarves, and those with congenital defects. Some camp inmates were used as subjects to train medical students in surgery. Jewish physicians in one camp surreptitiously recorded observations about the impact of starvation on the body.

The question of whether any of these activities carried out in the name of medical or scientific research upon unconsenting, coerced human beings deserves the label of *research* or *experimentation* is controversial (*see* Katz, this volume). When the description of research is broadened further to include the intentional killing of human beings in order to establish what methods are most efficient, references to "research" and "experimentation" begin to seem completely strained (*see* Kor, Konopka, and Vigorito, this volume). Injecting a half-starved, young girl with phenol to see how quickly she will die or trying out various forms of phosgene gas on camp inmates in the hope of finding cheap, clean, and efficient modes of killing so the state can effectively prosecute genocide is not the sort of activity associated with the term *research*. But murder and genocide are not the same as intentionally causing someone to suffer and die to fulfill a scientific goal. Killing for scientific purposes, while certainly as evil as murder in the service of racial hygiene, is, nonetheless, morally different. The torture and killing that were at the core of Nazi medical experiments involves not only torture and murder but also the exploitation of human beings to serve the goals of science. To describe what happened in language other than that of human experimentation blurs the nature of the wrong-doing. The evil inherent in Nazi medical experimentation was not simply that people suffered and died but that they were exploited for science and medicine as they died.

Isolating these crimes from the realm of biomedical experimentation is to draw a line that inappropriately weakens mainstream medicine and science's connection with dastardly acts (*see* Friedman, this volume). Doctors and scientists, many holding university and medical school appointments, did make men, women, and children suffer and die in the name of advancing knowledge in science and medicine.

The ethical issues raised by experimentation in the camps was forcefully brought to my attention by a physiologist, Robert Pozos, who was then in the department of physiology at the University of Minnesota in Duluth (*see* Pozos, this volume). At the end of a lecture I gave at the Duluth campus of the University of Minnesota in October, 1987, on the ethics of human experimentation, he asked my advice as to whether he should cite data in papers he intended to write on the effects of hypothermia, exposure to extremely cold temperatures, that had been obtained in a series of incredibly cruel inquiries using concentration camp inmates.

Pozos, an expert in the field of hypothermia, had been wrestling with this issue, as had others in the field of physiology, for many years.[18] When he raised the question with me about the ethics of using information from heinous experiments, I assumed that the data had not been cited previously in scientific literature. This assumption was false. The findings had been cited by dozens of scientists from many countries in numerous peer-reviewed publications. As I subsequently discovered, Pozos himself had previously cited the data. Nevertheless, it took courage for him to raise the question of the ethics of using this data. Many of Pozos' scientific peers and predecessors had simply ignored the moral issues involved and had cited the Nazi experiments on camp residents without comment or discussion. Pozos told me that the Nazi hypothermia research was widely known among experts in the physiology of exposure to cold temperatures in the US, Canada, Britain, Japan, and the Soviet Union. He also said there might be further information on the experiments stored in archives in Germany or elsewhere. Should these documents be found, would it be right for him or anyone else to examine them and publish their findings?

The experiments done in the concentration camps on hypothermia were undertaken to solve a problem of special importance to the German armed forces. In the first months of the war, German aviation and naval leaders were very concerned about the loss of pilots and seamen from exposure to cold. The theater of German military operations was rapidly expanding into cold areas of the globe such as Norway, the Baltic Sea, and the Soviet Union. The German military wanted to learn all they could about the ability of men to survive exposure to cold and about the best techniques for reviving them. The Luftwaffe especially wanted answers quickly since they were losing many highly trained, especially valuable pilots to cold exposure.

The military had turned to the medical branch of the Luftwaffe for answers. The military physicians felt that the best way to learn about the limits of human endurance to cold and techniques for revival was to conduct a series of experiments in which men would be exposed to cold temperatures under controlled conditions. At first, their discussions presumed the use of German military volunteers, but eventually it was decided that the fastest way to proceed was to use inmates in concentration camps. By exposing human beings to potentially lethal cold temperatures answers might be more readily available (*see* Pozos, this volume). However, the shift to exposures to lethal temperatures led the military to turn away from the use of volunteers in carefully controlled trials to the use of camp inmates who would be experimented upon under primitive and crude circumstances.

Two sets of experiments involving hypothermia were actually performed. The first set involved inmates at the Dachau concentration camp.[19] German military physicians from the physiology department at the University of Kiel came to the camp to supervise the experiments. They were concerned that the results be generalizable to Aryan men so they tried to select political prisoners and dissidents who were not Jews or Gypsies as their subjects.

The university physiologists worked under the supervision of SS physician Sigmund Rascher, who administered Dachau. He was a personal favorite of Heinrich Himmler, chief of the SS. Subjects were selected from among camp inmates with an eye toward their race, health, and age and then were fed an improved diet to make them more suitable subjects. After a few weeks, the men were brought to a special unit in the camp where a vat had been built containing ice and freezing water. The men were immersed until they became unconscious. Vital signs of those thus exposed were monitored and recorded. The suffering endured by the subjects was enormous. Various techniques were used to try and revive those who did not die. Those who did die were autopsied on the spot.

The physiologists from the University of Kiel were not comfortable working with Rascher, not because of the suffering of the subjects but because they doubted his scientific acumen. They conducted experiments on approximately 40 subjects and then left to write up their findings.

Rascher decided to continue the experiments on his own both to prove that he could conduct research worthy of an appointment to a university faculty and to curry favor with Himmler. At first, he continued to use the special facility that had been built, but later, he decided to simulate more natural conditions of cold exposure. In Rascher's experiments, men were kept standing outside at night while freezing cold water was periodically poured over them. Again, vital signs and temperatures were monitored. The suffering of those subjected to these tortures was so great that some of those involved in carrying out the research did not follow their orders. Conditions outdoors varied a great deal, and the subjects involved were in far worse physical condition than those who had been subjected to the first series of experiments.

Both sets of experiments were cruel, inhumane, and immoral. Those involved suffered a great deal. About one-quarter of the subjects died. Their suffering was so great that some of those who assisted in the experiments tried to take action to help the subjects, thereby casting doubt over the reliability of the findings that were reported (*see* Berger, this volume). Nonetheless, the researchers believed that the information they obtained, at least in the first series of experiments, was accurate and valid. The findings were presented at a meeting of military physicians in Berlin. The German armed forces apparently used the findings in the design of survival suits for soldiers and in developing resuscitation policies for those exposed to cold temperatures (*see* Pozos, this vol).

Pozos believed and continues to believe (*see* Pozos and Katz, this vol) that the findings produced by the hypothermia studies are of scientific value. Other experts in hypothermia agree.[18] Pozos and some other physiologists believe that these studies are the only source of information concerning both the response of the body to prolonged extremes of cold temperature under conditions of total immersion and of the efficacy and reliability of certain resuscitation techniques.

Pozos' question about whether it is ethical to use information from Nazi hypothermia inquiries came hard on the heels of a similar question about a different set of Nazi experiments. Scientists working for a private firm under contract to the US Government's Environmental Protection Agency had submitted a report about the dangers of phosgene gas to the agency. The report included references to work that German scientists had conducted in various concentration camps to determine the killing powers of phosgene gas. When some EPA scientists objected to any references to Nazi research appearing in a government-sponsored report, the director of the EPA, Lee Thomas, decided to delete them.

In both the hypothermia and phosgene gas examples, questions arise as to the morality of citing information obtained from experiments on unconsenting victims, many of whom died in the course of the experiments. The information was felt to have some validity by reputable scientists. The information was also seen as unique and difficult to obtain from other sources. The stakes in both the hypothermia and phosgene gas cases were set very high: Lives hung in the balance, depending on whether the results of the Nazi work were cited.

One line of response to the issue of citing Nazi data is to shed doubt on their validity (*see* Berger, this vol).[3] And there are many reasons to doubt that the findings of the hypothermia studies and the phosgene gas research are either valid or the only source of life-saving information. But in another sense, haggling over the merits of the methodology of Nazi science misses a more important point. Some experts not only believe the data in the hypothermia and phosgene gas studies are valid; they have long been referenced in biomedical literature. The results of these cruel inquiries were discovered and studied by scientists and doctors working for the armed forces of the US, Britain, and the Soviet Union at the conclusion of World War II. Reports, some classified, others not, were prepared using the information the Nazi scientists had obtained on the hypothermia research that was of special interest to the military for much the same reason the Wehrmacht and Luftwaffe had sought the data.

A summary report prepared for the American military about the hypothermia experiments has been cited in the peer-reviewed literature of medicine more than two dozen times since the end of World War II, most recently in a physiology textbook published in 1989. Not only were the data examined and referenced, but they were applied. British air–sea rescue experts used the Nazi data to modify rescue techniques for those exposed to cold water.[20] The force of the question "Should the data be used?" is diminished not only because there are reasons to doubt the reliability and exclusivity of the data but also because the question has already been answered: Nazi data have been used by many scientists from many nations.

There is another moral issue that does not hinge on the answer to the question of whether the research was well-designed or whether the findings are of enduring scientific value. How did physicians and scientists convince themselves that murderous experimentation was morally justified?

No one understood the need for justification more clearly than the doctors and scientists put on trial for their crimes after the conclusion of the war. The defendants admitted that dangerous and even lethal experiments had been conducted on unconsenting persons in prisons and other institutions. Some protested attempts by the prosecution, in its effort to highlight the barbarity of what they had done, to demean or disparage the caliber of their research. No one apologized for their role in various experiments conducted in the camps. Instead, those put on trial attempted to explain and justify what they had done, often couching their defense in explicitly moral terms.

The Ethics of Evil

Probably the most succinct precis of the moral arguments brought forward by physicians, public health officials, and scientists in defense of their participation both in experimentation in the concentration camps and in the "final solution" can be found in the transcripts of the Nuremberg trials. The first group of individuals to be put on trial by the Allies were physicians and public health officials. The role they had played in conducting or tolerating cruel and often lethal experiments in the camps dominated the trials.[47] As it happens, the same arguments that were brought forward in defense of the camp experiments were also used to justify participation in mass murder and attempts at the forced sterilization of camp inmates. A review of the major moral arguments presented by defendants at the Nuremberg trials sheds light not only on the moral rationales that were given for the hypothermia and phosgene gas experiments but also for the involvement of biomedicine in the broad sweep of what the prosecution termed "crimes against humanity."

Beginning the process of analyzing the moral defense of those who stood trial, aside from its intrinsic importance, is also an essential step in the assessment of the appropriateness and inappropriateness of references and analogies to the Holocaust in current bioethical debates.

One of the most common moral rationales given at the trials was that no wrong had been done because those who were subjects had volunteered. Prisoners might be freed, some defendants argued, if they survived the experiments. The prospects of release and pardon were mentioned very frequently during the trial since they were the basis for the claim that people participated voluntarily in the experiments.[19] On this line of thinking, experimentation was justified because it might actually benefit the subjects.

The major flaw with this moral rationale is simply that it was false. In 1989, the British newspaper, the *London Sun-*

day Observer, found a man who had survived the hypothermia experiments, which involved prolonged submersion in tanks of freezing water. The man now lives in Belgium. He had been sent to Dachau because of his political beliefs. He said that the researchers told him that if he survived the hypothermia experiments and then the decompression experiments, he might be freed. He was not. He said no prisoners were. However, he was given a medal by the Reich on the recommendation of the experimenters. The medal was given in recognition of the contributions he had made to medical science!

Granted, Nazi researchers did not keep their promises. But what if they had? Would arduous, even potentially lethal experimentation be justified by the promise of freedom if the subject survived the research? The answer to this position clearly seems to be no. It seems extremely coercive to tell a condemned prisoner that his only chance at freedom or even survival is to survive an arduous experiment. Consent means nothing where such an offer is concerned. Moreover, it seems immoral to even accept the offer of participation in painful, disabling, and potentially lethal experimentation as legitimate.

Another of the key rationales on the part of those put on trial was that only people who were doomed to die were used for biomedical purposes.[19] Time and again the doctors who froze screaming subjects to death or watched their brains explode as a result of rapid decompression stated that only prisoners condemned to death were used. It seemed morally defensible to physicians and scientists to learn from what they saw as the inevitable deaths of camp inmates.

This line of argument does not lack contemporary advocates. Jack Kevorkian, who rocketed to fame as the man who assisted Janet Adkins in committing suicide in the back of his Volkswagon van in a suburban Detroit campground, has long advocated dispatching prisoners condemned to die in such a way that we can either use them for research or obtain their organs and tissues to transplant to others. Prisoners, who are currently prohibited in some American states from participating in anything more than nontrivial medical research, have sued for the right to participate in riskier medical trials.

But putting aside the immoral grounds for condemning Jews, Gypsies, POWs, and others to death, are those who are condemned to die fair game for biomedical experimentation? The answer would seem to be no if only because even the condemned are not to be treated as mere instruments. Indeed, the very justification of the morality of capital punishment depends on the treatment of those who are doomed to die as more than things or objects.

A third ethical rationale for performing brutal experiments upon innocent subjects was that participation in lethal research offered expiation to the subjects. By being injected, frozen, or transplanted subjects could cleanse themselves of their crimes. Suffering prior to death as a way to atone for sin seemed to be a morally acceptable rationale for causing suffering to those who were guilty of crimes.

The problem with this ethical defense is that those who were experimented on or made to suffer by German physicians and scientists were never guilty of any crime other than that of belonging to a despised ethnic or racial minority or for holding unacceptable political views. Even if those who were experimented upon or killed had been guilty of some serious crime, would it have been moral to use medical experimentation or the risk of death as a form of punishment or expiation? It is hard to see how these goals square with the goals of medicine or health care. It is impossible to see how such a position is persuasive with respect to incompetent persons and minor children.

A fourth moral rationale, one that is especially astounding even by the standards of self-delusion in evidence throughout the trial proceedings, was that scientists and physicians had to act in a value-neutral manner. To use a philosophical description, some of those who had tortured, maimed, and killed pled logical positivism in their defense. Although they did not actually use these words, they maintained that scientists and doctors are not responsible for and have no expertise about values and thus could not be held accountable for their actions.

> ...if the experiment is ordered by the state, this moral responsibility of experimenter toward the experimental subject relates to the way in which the experiment is performed, not the experiment itself.[19] (p. 542)

Some researchers only felt themselves responsible for the proper design and conduct of their research. They felt no moral responsibility for what had occurred in the camps because they did not have any expertise concerning moral matters. They claimed to have left decisions about these matters to others.

The view that scientists must leave moral matters to others has some resonance in contemporary debates about medicine and science. But there are few who would argue that physicians or scientists have immunity for the consequences of their actions simply because they are not experts in values. Most people are not professors of religion, law, or philosophy, and yet, we hold each other accountable for our actions.

The fifth moral justification for what happened presented by many of the defendants was that they had done what they did for the defense and security of their country. All actions were done to preserve the Reich during "total" war.[19]

> Germany was engaged in war at that time. Millions of soldiers had to give up their lives because they were called upon to fight by the state. The state employed the civilian population for work according to state requirements. The state ordered employment in chemical factories which was detrimental to health.

> ...In the same way the state ordered the medical men to make experiments with new weapons against dangerous diseases.[19]

Total war, in which the survival of the nation hangs in the balance, justifies exceptions to ordinary morality, the defendants maintained. Those who had run the camps, made the selections on the ramps, and had conducted war-related research had done so at the legitimate request of state authorities. They had followed legitimate orders from legitimate authorities in order to preserve their nation. Allied prosecutors had much to ponder in thinking about this defense in light of the fire-bombing of Dresden and Tokyo and the dropping of nuclear bombs on Hiroshima and Nagasaki.

Arguments about what total war permits in terms of morality raised tough issues for the Allied prosecutors and continue to raise hard questions for us now. Those who build or might fire nuclear weapons must confront the issue on a daily basis. However, none of the issues in contemporary bioethics that so often elicit analogies to Nazism—genetic engineering, fetal tissue research, abortion, or euthanasia—have a plausible connection to rationales concerning the rights of the state to compel behavior in times of war. Whatever the motives and moral thinking are of those who perform abortions or terminate medical care, the requirements of total war play no role and thus have no analogy to this aspect of Nazi conduct.

The last rationale is the one that appears to carry the most weight among all the moral defenses offered. Many who conducted lethal experiments or actively engaged in genocide argued that it was reasonable to sacrifice the interests of the few in order to benefit the majority.

The most distinguished of the scientists who was put on trial, Gerhard Rose, the head of the Koch Institute of Tropical Medicine in Berlin, said that he initially opposed performing potentially lethal experiments to create a vaccine for typhus on camp inmates. But he came to believe that it made no sense not to risk the lives of 100 or 200 men in pursuit of a vaccine when 1000 men a day were dying of typhus on the Eastern front. What, he asked, were the deaths of 100 men compared to the possible benefit of getting a prophylactic vaccine capable of saving tens of thousands? Rose, because he admitted that he had anguished about his own moral duty when asked by the Wehrmacht to perform the typhus experiments in a concentration camp, raises the most difficult and most plausible moral argument in defense of lethal experimentation.

The prosecution encountered some difficulty with Rose's argument. The defense team for Rose noted that the Allies themselves justified the compulsory drafting of men for military service throughout the war, knowing many would certainly die, on the grounds that the sacrifice of the few to save the many was morally just. Moreover, they also pointed out that throughout history medical researchers in Western countries used versions of utilitarianism to justify dangerous experiments on prisoners and institutionalized persons.

Justifying the sacrifice of the few to benefit the majority is a position that must be taken seriously as a moral argument. However, in the context of the Nazi regime, it is fair to point out that sacrifice was not born equally by all as is true of a compulsory draft that allows no exceptions. It is also true that many would argue that no degree of benefit should permit intrusions into certain fundamental rights.

Crude utilitarianism is a position that sometimes rears its head in contemporary bioethical debate. Some argue that we ought not spend scarce social resources on certain groups within our society such as the elderly so that other groups, such as children, may have greater benefits. Those who want to invoke the Nazi analogy may be able to show that this form of crude utilitarian thinking does motivate some of the policies or actions taken by contemporary biomedical scientists and health care professionals.

In closely reviewing the statements that accompany the six major moral rationales for murder, torture, and mutilation conducted in the camps—freedom was a possible benefit, only the condemned were used, expiation was a possible benefit, a lack of moral expertise, the need to preserve the state in conditions of total war, and the morality of sacrificing a few to benefit many—it becomes clear that the conduct of those who worked in the concentration camps was sometimes guided by moral rationales. These positions need to be understood and critically assessed if we are to clearly understand the values that allowed biomedical scientists and health care professionals to participate in inhumane experimentation and genocide.

It is also clear that all of these moral arguments were nested within a biomedical interpretation of the danger facing Germany. Time and again the physicians and public health officials at the trials refer to the threat posed by "inferior races" and "useless eaters" to the welfare of the Reich. The paradigm of the state metaphorically facing a biological threat to its overall well-being that could only be alleviated by the kind of medical interventions doctors would use to fight disease within the body is reflected in the medical literature and training of health care professionals both before and during the war.[2,5,6]

Physicians could justify their actions, whether direct involvement with euthanasia and lethal experiments, or merely support for Hitler and the Reich, on the grounds that Jews, homosexuals, the congenitally handicapped, and Slavs posed a threat, a biological threat, a genetic threat, to the existence and future of the Reich. The appropriate response to such a threat was to eliminate it, just as a physician must eliminate a burst appendix by means of surgery or a dangerous bacteria using penicillin.

Viewing specific ethnic groups and populations as threatening the health of the German state permitted and in the view of those on trial, demanded the involvement of medicine in mass genocide, sterilization, and lethal experimentation. The biomedical paradigm provided the theoretical basis for allowing those sworn to the Hippocratic principle of nonmaleficence to kill in the name of the state.

The Neglect of the Holocaust
and Nazism in Bioethics

Why has the field of bioethics not attended more closely
to the Holocaust and the role played by German medicine
and science in the Holocaust? Why have the moral arguments
bluntly presented by the Nazis received so little attention?
These are questions that do not admit simple answers.

The crimes of doctors and biomedical scientists revealed
at the Nuremberg trials were overwhelming in their cruelty.
Physicians and scientists supervised and in some cases,
actively participated in the genocide of millions, directly
engaged in the torture of thousands, and provided the scientific underpinning for genocide. Hundreds of thousands of
psychiatric patients and senile elderly persons were killed
under the direct supervision of physicians and nurses. Numerous scientists and physicians, some of whom headed internationally renowned research centers and hospitals, engaged
in cruel and sometimes lethal experiments on unconsenting
inmates of concentration camps.

Ironically, the scale of immorality is one of the reasons
why the moral reasoning of health care professionals and
biomedical scientists during the Nazi era has received little
attention from contemporary bioethics scholars. It is clear
that what Nazi doctors, biologists, and public health officials
did was immoral. The indisputable occurrence of wrong-
doing suggests that there is little for the ethicist to say
except to join with others in condemnation of what happened.
But condemnation is not sufficient. After all, many of those
who committed crimes did so firm in their belief in the moral
rectitude of their actions. Whereas bioethics cannot be held
accountable for every horrible act that a physician chooses
to explain by using moral terms, those who teach bioethics
in the hope that it can effect conduct or character must come
to terms with the fact that biomedicine's role in the Holocaust was frequently defended on moral grounds.

Guilt by association has also played a role in making
some bioethicists shy away from closely examining what

medicine and science did during the Nazi era. Many doctors and scientists who were contemporaries of those put on trial at Nuremberg denied any connection between their own work or professional identities and those of the defendants. Contemporary doctors and scientists are, understandably, even quicker to deny any connection between what Nazi doctors or scientists did and their own activities or conduct. Many scholars and health care professionals, in condemning the crimes committed in the name of medicine and the biomedical sciences during the Holocaust, insist that all those who perpetrated those crimes were aberrant, deviant, atypical representatives of the health and scientific professions. Placing these acts and those who did them on the fringe of biomedicine keeps a needed distance between then and now.

To suggest that the men and women currently engaged in research on the human genome or in transplanting fetal tissue obtained from elective abortions are immoral monsters on a par with a Josef Mengele or a Karl Brandt is to miss the crucial point that the Nazis carried out genocide for moral reasons and from a biological world view that has little connection with the values that motivate contemporary biomedical physicians and scientists. Abortion may or may not be a morally defensible act, but it is a different act from injecting a Jewish baby with gasoline in order to preserve the racial purity of the Reich. Scholars in bioethics may have avoided any analysis of Nazi medicine simply because they feared the wrath of those who felt belittled, insulted, or falsely accused by any connection being drawn between their behavior and that of Nazi doctors, nurses, and scientists. Yet, by saying little and thereby allowing all Nazi scientists and doctors to be transformed into madmen or monsters, bioethicists ignore the fact that the Germany of the first half of this century was one of the most "civilized," technologically advanced, and scientifically sophisticated societies on the face of the globe. In medicine and biology, pre World War II Germany could easily hold its own with any other scientifically literate society of the day. Indeed, the crimes carried out by doctors and scientists during the tenure of the Third Reich are all the more staggering in their impact and are all the more difficult to interpret precisely because Germany was such a technologically and scientifically advanced society.

The Holocaust is the exemplar of evil in our century. The medical crimes of that time stand as the clearest examples available of moral wrong-doing in biomedical science. Bioethics may have been silent precisely because there seems to be nothing to say about an unparalleled biomedical immorality, but silence leads to omission. By saying little about the most horrific crimes ever carried out in the name of biomedicine and the moral views that permitted these crimes to be done, bioethics contributes to allowing these events to fade away from the history of biomedicine and bioethics.

Appendix[21]

Science and Medicine in Nazi Germany

A Chronological Overview

1896	Alfred Ploetz publishes *Grundlinien einer Rassenhygiene* introducing the concept of "racial hygiene" into German medicine. The psychologist Alfred Jost publishes *Das Recht auf den Tod* in which he argues that the state is justified in killing incurably ill mental patients.
1913	Eugen Fischer, an anatomist at Freiburg University, publishes a book about mixed-blood people in Southwest Africa, recommending that they be offered minimal protection only "as a race inferior to ourselves."
1917–1918	Patients in German psychiatric hospitals are given low priority in the government's wartime rationing scheme. Roughly half of them die as a result of starvation.
1918	Hermann Siemens publishes a booklet, "What is Race Hygiene?," in which he warns that the

quality of the human race will decline if the genetically unfit are allowed to breed more than the fit.

1920   Alfred Hoche, professor of psychiatry, and Rudolf Binding, a professor of law, publish a book, *Die Freigabe der Vernichtung Lebensunwerten Lebens* (Permission for the Extermination of Lives Not Worth Living). They hold that the right to life must be earned and justified, not assumed. Those incapable of human feeling—"empty human husks" in the mental hospitals—should be destroyed as a humane act.

1923   Hitler, while imprisoned, reads a textbook, *Outline of Human Genetics and Racial Hygiene*, and incorporates some of its ideas into *Mein Kampf*. Two of the book's authors are Fischer and Fritz Lenz.

1927   The Kaiser-Wilhelm-Gesellschaft, the most important institution for promoting the study of science in Germany, sets up an Institute of Anthropology, Human Heredity, and Eugenics in Berlin. Its director is Fischer, who becomes chairman two years later of the committee on racial crosses of the International Federation of Eugenic Organizations (whose president is an American).

1929   Forty-two male and two female physicians form the National Socialist Physicians' League to coordinate Nazi medical policy and "to purify the German medical community of the influence of Jewish Bolshevism."

Nearly 15,000 persons have been involuntarily sterilized in the US during the past 20 years, mainly prisoners and those in homes for the mentally ill.

Nazi party creates an institute at Alt-Rehse near Berlin to educate physicians in the ideology of the party.

1931   Lenz publishes the third edition of his widely read textbook on human genetics in which he terms National Socialism "applied biology."

1931   The University of Erlangen's general student committee asks that a chair of race-investigations, race-science, race-hygiene, and genetics be set up.

Dec. 1931   Himmler orders that members of the SS must obtain permission—to be granted on grounds of hereditary and racial health—to marry. Lenz calls this "a worthwhile exercise."

July 1932   The Prussian State Health Council recommends enacting a law to permit the "voluntary" sterilization of schizophrenics, manic-depressives, congenital epileptics, and those with other congenital mental defects.

1932   More than 20 institutes for racial science and racial hygiene have been established at German universities. At least 10 journals are being published on the subject of racial hygiene.

Jan., 1933   Twenty eight hundred doctors, or 6% of the whole medical profession, have joined the Nazi Physicians' League. This is three times the rate for the general population and 15 times higher than the number of judges who have joined. Hitler comes to power.

April, 1933   Law passed requiring the dismissal of all Jews and half Jews from state employment.

June 2, 1933   Law passed dismissing the right to practice in social medical system if physician is of non-Aryan origin or was a member of the communist or socialist party.

July 14, 1933 — Law for the Prevention of Genetically Diseased Offspring passed. Permits sterilization of anyone suffering from "genetically determined" illnesses, including feeblemindedness, deafness, blindness, severe alcoholism, Huntington's Disease, schizophrenia, severe malformations, and insanity.

July, 1933 — Concentration camps established by Goering in Berlin and Himmler in Dachau for "enemies of the state."

1934 — One hundered and eighty one Genetic Health courts and Appellate Genetic Health courts established to administer the Law for the Prevention of Genetically Diseased Offspring. Doctors required to register all genetic defectives and to undergo training in genetic pathology.

Arthur Gutt, Ernst Rudin, and Falk Ruttke publish a commentary on the law *Gesetz zur Verhuting erkranken Nachwuchses vom 14.7.1933*. They argue that the law "should be seen as a clean break with the debris and faintheartedness of an outmoded worldview and the exaggerated suicidal compassion of past centuries." They maintain that it is not just the cost of caring for the mentally ill and those with hereditary illness that justifies the law but also the threat to the social system and moral principles that the further unchecked breeding of these groups portends.

March, 1935 — Fischer and Lenz, with other doctors and civil servants, discuss the sterilization of the "Rhineland bastards," mixed-race offspring resulting from the occupation of the Rhineland after World War I by French colonial troops from Africa.

Sept.–Nov., 1935 So-called Nuremberg Laws passed that exclude Jews from citizenship and prohibit marriage or sexual intercourse between Jews and citizens of German or related blood. All prospective marriage partners are to be examined by a physician to prevent "racial pollution."

Nov., 1936   Psychiatrist Robert Ritter starts a study to identify and trace movements of Gypsies in Germany.

Spring, 1937   Sterilizations of "Rhineland bastards" carried out.

Oct., 1937   Otmar von Verschuer, professor of anthropology and racial hygiene at Frankfurt (and a physician), protests to the Minister of Justice that his expert opinion in a "race-dishonor" case—in which he had concluded that a defendant was a half-Jew—had been rejected by a court.

March, 1938   Karl Kleist, professor of psychiatry at Frankfurt, reports on the mental hospital at Herborn. It was one of several where the killing of patients through hunger and untreated illness had become established policy. His report ends:

                    "As long as there is no law 'for the destruction of lives unworthy to be lived', those who are beyond cure have the right to humane treatment which assures their continued existence. Expenditure on these unfortunates should not be allowed to fall below a certain minimum level."

                    Some time later, five professors of psychiatry, with Lenz, some SS doctors and medical civil servants, draft a law to permit the killing of psychiatric patients.

                    American Medical Association rejects request from 5000 black physicians to join the association.

The AMA refusal is widely reported in German medical journals.

June, 1939 — In a lecture, Fischer says:

"When a people wants, somehow or other, to preserve its own nature, it must reject alien racial elements, and when these have already insinuated themselves, it must suppress and eliminate them. The Jew is such an alien and, therefore, when he wants to insinuate himself, he must be warded off. This is self-defence. In saying this, I do not characterize every Jew as inferior, as Negroes are, and I do not underestimate the greatest enemy with whom we have to fight. But I reject Jewry with every means in my power, and without reserve, in order to preserve the hereditary endowment of my people."

Interior Minister Wilhelm Frick orders all twins born in the Reich to be registered with public health offices for purposes of genetic research.

Aug. 31, 1939 — Sterilizations largely come to an end. Best estimates are that 350,000–400,000 were performed, with 2000 persons dying as a result of postoperative complications.

Sept. 1, 1939 — Poland invaded and World War II begins. *SS Einsatzgruppen* ordered to find and kill all potential Polish leaders and intellectuals. "Resettlement of 'alien' elements" (mainly Jews) outside of German ethnic space into ghettoes on grounds of racial purity begins.

Oct., 1939 — Hitler issues order allowing German doctors to perform involuntary mercy killings (*gnadentod*) of patients judged incurably ill.

Polish mental patients gassed at Posen by occupying German army.

Federal Board for the Scientific Registration of Hereditary or Other Severe Congenital Diseases created. All doctors and midwives required to register birth of all deformed children.

Euthanasia program for mentally ill adults starts (orders creating program are backdated to coincide with start of war). Specially designated physicians examine questionnaires returned by mental hospitals on each patient. A Charitable Ambulance Service is created to transport patients to the State Mental Hospitals Association sites where killing is done. Nine professors of psychiatry and 39 other doctors in panels of four process 283,000 questionnaires. They mark at least 75,000 with a cross, signifying that the patient is to be gassed. Gassing is done in rooms built to resemble showers to calm victims.

Expert panels of three doctors formed to make judgments about euthanasia for severely disabled newborns. Experts read the medical report from the local doctor, and if a negative decision is reached, drugs are used to kill children. More than 20 children's departments are established in hospitals for this purpose. Approximately 5000 children, some as old as 17, are killed by the end of the war.

Jan., 1940   First experiments conducted by physicians at Brandenburg Hospital to find optimal gas for mass killing.

June, 1941   USSR invaded (Operation Barbarossa). In July, "special action groups" begin mass shootings of Jews, Gypsies, and mental patients.

Aug., 1941   By this date, 70,000 mental patients have been killed in Germany. Gassing is stopped in part because of public disquiet and protests of some churchmen. "Covert" or "wild" euthanasia of mentally ill and retarded begins using starvation, drugs, and neglect. Another 70,000 patients are killed during the next four years.

Sept., 1941   First experiments, under control of physicians, in using Zyklon B (hydrocyanic acid) to kill Russian prisoners of war at Auschwitz.

Oct., 1941   Planning begins for creating extermination camp at Belzec (Poland). Some of the doctors and nurses who worked in the euthanasia program for the mentally ill and their equipment are moved to Poland. Killing by gunshot or lethal injection of mental patients in Riga, Minsk, and Kiev begins.

Jan., 1942   Friedrich Mennecke, a physician involved in the euthanasia program, takes a group of doctors and nurses to set up an extermination center at Chelmno for Polish Jews and Gypsies.

Jan. 20, 1942   Wannsee Conference (Berlin): Conference on the Final Solution of the Jewish Question. Himmler announces the policy of "Vernichtung Durch Arbeit"—Extermination Through Work.

March, 1942   Mass gassings begin at Belzec and Mauthausen (start of Operation Reinhard, the systematic destruction of Polish Jews by gassing).

April, 1942   Wolfgang Abel, a department head at the Berlin Institute of Anthropology, gives a prestigious lecture in which he warns that there are only two possible responses to the racial threat posed by the Soviet Union "either the extermination of the Russian people or Germanization of its Nordic elements." (Approximately 3,000,000 Russian prisoners of war were eventually killed.)

May 20, 1942   High-altitude decompression "experiments" completed by Sigmund Rascher with supervision of Luftwaffe at Dachau.

July, 1942   Resettlement begins of hundreds of thousands of Polish Jews, "useless eaters," to Treblinka, Auschwitz, and other camps for killing.

July, 1942   Mutilating "experiments" initiated on women in Ravensbruck concentration camp to test effectiveness of drugs against gunshot and other simulated battlefield injuries.

Aug., 1942   Hypothermia experiments begun by Rascher and University of Kiel Professors at Dachau.

Oct. 26, 1942   Data on hypothermia studies presented at annual meeting of Luftwaffe medical service in Nuremberg. There were 95 physicians in attendance.

Nov. 30, 1942   Bavarian Ministry of the Interior issues special rules for feeding mentally ill. Those who worked "effectively should get more and better food than those who did not work." Hundreds of patients are then starved to death.

Dec., 1942   A department head at the Institute of Brain Research, Hallervorden reports that he has been able during the year to dissect the brains of 500 feeble-minded individuals from the extermination center in Brandenburg.

                Carl Schneider, professor of psychiatry at Heidelberg, sets up a research ward in Wiesloch mental hospital. Idiots and epileptics are to be physiologically and psychologically assessed. After being killed at another nearby mental hospital, their brains are dissected and studied.

                Data from hypothermia studies presented at conference of Wehrmacht physicians in Berlin.

Feb. 18, 1943   A small group of medical students at the University of Munich, founders in late 1941 of the "White Rose" resistance organization, are arrested as enemies of the Reich. They are subsequently excecuted.

March 1943   Ritter reports to the public health office that he has identified 21,500 persons as Gypsies using his system of racial classification.

Himmler issues order that only physicians with training in anthropology can make selections among concentration camp inmates as to who should live and who should die.

May, 1943   Results of Ravensbruck experiments reported at Congress of Reich Physicians. Awards given to researchers by German Orthopedic Society. Hypothermia findings reported to a select group of physicians at a meeting in Berlin including Ferdinand Sauerbruch, chief of surgery at the University of Berlin.

March, 1944   Hallervorden reports: "I have received 697 brains in all, including those which I took out myself in Brandenburg." (Part of this collection was kept at the University of Frankfurt until 1989.)

Aug., 1944   The last of the Gypsies, who were confirmed as such by Ritter's work, are killed in Auschwitz.

Throughout 1944, Mengele is sending "scientific" material to the Institute of Anthropology in Berlin. The material includes eyes from murdered Gypsies, internal organs from murdered children, and sera from twins deliberately infected with typhoid.

Experiments begun with help of H. Eppinger to develop potable water from seawater. Control group receives no water for 12 days; all die.

Sept., 1944 August Hirt of the University of Strasbourg orders his skull and skeletal collection of "Jewish Bolshevik commisars" and other racial "inferiors" destroyed for fear they will fall into the hands of advancing allied troops.

Mental patients in Bavaria are killed to make beds available for war casualties. Responsibility for selecting and killing patients left to individual doctors in mental hospitals.

May, 1945 The war ends. Only 15% of the patients in mental hospitals at the start of the war have survived. More than 38,000 physicians, almost half of all doctors in Germany, had joined the Nazi party. More than 7% of all physicians were members of the *SS*, compared with less than 0.5% of the general population.

July, 1945 US soldiers discover that killing of mental patients has continued in a hospital near Kaufbeuren in Bavaria.

1946 Lenz is appointed professor of human genetics at the University of Gottingen.

von Verschuer continues as professor of human genetics at the University of Munster. Fischer continues to edit various scholarly journals. Hallervorden continues as department head at the Institute of Brain Research.

1949 Two German physicians, Alexander Mitscherlich and Fred Mielke, publish a book on the the Nuremberg medical trials. Ten thousand copies are sent to the West German Physicians' Association for free distribution; none are distributed. No single mention of the book appears in German medical literature for the next two decades.

1959 Albert Hegnauer writes in the Annals of the New York Academy of Sciences that one of the two most important sources of information on lethal limits of hypothermia are "experiments conducted at Dachau during World War II."

1973   Falk Foundation creates an international prize in gastroenterology in honor of Eppinger.

1976   Commemorative stamp issued in West Germany in honor of Ferdinand Sauerbruch, one of Germany's most renowned surgeons in the 1930s and 1940s and a supporter of the Nazi regime.

Spring, 1980   Some German medical students and physicians organize an unofficial meeting at the time of the official West German medical society annual meeting at which the issue of medicine under the Nazis is discussed for the first time in West Germany.

1988   Scientists under contract in the pollution assessment branch of the EPA cite phosgene gas studies conducted by Nazis in preparing risk assessment of the environmental impact of the gas.

1989   It is revealed that skeletal and tissue samples from Holocaust victims are being used for teaching purposes at various medical schools in West Germany.

At least 45 research articles in peer-reviewed medical and scientific literature have cited various experiments conducted by Nazis in concentration camps. Many are in the field of hypothermia research. A leading American-British textbook on high-altitude physiology cites Leo Alexander's report prepared at the end of the War on the hypothermia experiments among its references without comment on or clarification of the source of information.

1990   In the face of rising international concern, a
             number of German medical schools and
             institutes bury their tissue sample collections
             including the Hallervorden collection dating
             from the war years since they may include the
             remains of Holocaust victims.

             Memorial erected at the site where tissue
             specimens obtained from Holocaust victims
             were buried at the University of Tubingen is
             desecrated.

From: *When Medicine Went Mad* Ed.: A. Caplan
©1992 The Humana Press Inc.

The Use of Information from Nazi "Experiments"

The Case of Hypothermia

Scientific Inquiry and Ethics

The Dachau Data

Robert S. Pozos

Introduction

During World War II, lethal biomedical experiments were performed on nonconsenting human subjects in Nazi Germany. The data from these experiments have been referenced numerous times in scientific literature. This paper will present the scientific and ethical arguments as to whether the information gathered in the concentration camps should continue to be referenced in the scientific literature. The publishing of these experiments and their subsequent referencing bring centerstage the question of the relationship between scientific inquiry and ethics.

Since the time of Aristotle, scientific inquiry was considered to be separate from the discipline of ethics.[1] There seems to be a natural difference between these two schools of thought in that scientific inquiry's ultimate goal is to arrive at principles that describe certain physical phenomenon. Ethics, on the other hand, is a discipline that does not have a final resolution since it is constantly changing. For example, the law of gravity is a general physical principle that is valid for most physical situations. On the other hand, the commandment *Thou shall not kill* is an ethical principle that is not always constant since it is acknowledged that killing in self-defense is permissible. However, most results of scientific inquiry in the biological sciences are not as pure as one would like to believe since biological data are conditioned by the experiment. For example, the anesthetics that are used in an experiment, the preparation of the biological material, and so forth all will influence the findings of the experiment. Nevertheless, ethics and scientific inquiry coexist. The question is whether they should be integrated.

The integration of ethics and scientific inquiry is by nature difficult. Instead of grappling with the relationship between these dissimilar disciplines, one solution is not to have an integration. This approach would entirely disregard ethical considerations and let science develop the solutions to its questions. The consequence of this approach is that it would eventually lead to some form of society in which practical solutions to problems are considered good for the well being of society.[2,3] Eventually, this form of thinking would lead to a utilitarian society in which the individual would have no rights.

A partial solution to this quandary in which ethics and scientific inquiry seem to have different end points is to perform a case-by-case analysis. This approach might yield guidelines that allow one to evaluate data by their scientific and ethical significance and then decide on their implementation and dissemination. It is important to emphasize that these guidelines should not stifle scientific inquiry and also should not allow it to go unchecked at the expense of compromising humanity.

The experiments conducted by the Nazis in Dachau during World War II and their subsequent publishing and referencing are used as an example to study the relationship between scientific inquiry and ethics. This example is used because there is adequate information to study the Nazi's scientific principles, methods, and data and their subsequent evaluation and referencing of this data by other scientists.

Before the relationship between scientific inquiry and ethics can be addressed, it is necessary to evaluate the information as to its accuracy and further, whether the researchers involved were aware of the basic priniciples underlying scientific inquiry.[4] In this fashion, the various arguments will focus on the continued reference of unethically gathered valid information. Most discussions regarding ethical use or misuse of research results deal with data that are falsified or plagiarized. Obviously, in those cases, there is no reason to reference that information. The consequences might be different, however, if the information is valid.

These experiments were conducted during a particularly tragic period in scientific history when physician–scientists were involved in the generation of information gathered from human subjects, some of whom were deliberately killed during the experiments. This dark chapter in research has been used to study the various social-political forces that were conducive for scientists to design and execute unethical experiments[5] in the name of national survival or national philosophy.[6]

Rationale of Experiments

During World War II, Nazi Germany faced a number of technical questions concerning human performance in various hostile environments and consequently, supported a wide range of experiments on human subjects. Because of the wide scope of biomedical experiments that were performed by German scientists, this chapter will concentrate only on the hypothermia experiments that were a continuation of the high-altitude studies. The Germans, British, and Americans were developing planes that could fly at high altitudes. A consequence of air combat and air campaigns was that pilots were shot down and landed in cold water. In addition, the German Navy was losing a large number of personnel in the cold North Sea. There were no data available to document how long the downed pilots could survive in the frigid North Sea. The solution to these questions, as well as others, was considered important by certain groups of Nazi administrators and scientists.[7,8] From a historical point of view, at that time, the number of papers that had been published that dealt with human response to cold water and/or air was very limited. In short, there was a dearth of information available concerning physiological responses to the cold that was directly applicable to the treatment of the hypothermic downed pilot in the North Sea.[9] In addition, there was no current information available as to the efficacy of various rewarming strategies. Equally challenging was the fact that hypothermic individuals would sometimes die when they were safely on board after being rescued.[10] According to some, therefore, the German scientists were seeking answers to "legitimate scientific goals."[11]

The Experiments

The following account is based on the report submitted by Leo Alexander, a major in the US Army Medical Corps who analyzed the secret written records that had been submitted to Heinrich Himmler by Nazi physician–scientists and that had been found buried in a cave in Germany.[12] The cache of information was discovered by American troops and became part of the Nuremberg documents used in the prosecution of Nazi war criminals. Alexander's report of the experiments conducted in Nazi Germany is one that is frequently referenced.

During World War II, Weltz, a physiologist, was interested in determining the most beneficial way to rewarm hypothermic animals. He discovered that he could rewarm severely hypothermic animals by immersing them in warm water of 40°C (104°F). If the water was warmer than 40°C, more animals survived. Another investigator, Lutz, used large adult pigs and was able to confirm the results of Weltz's work on guinea pigs. Since it was acknowledged that neither group of animals has similar temperature-regulating abilities to humans, Sigmond Rascher petitioned Himmler to administer a series of experiments on prisoners of war to substantiate the animal experiments.[11,13] Rascher had recently codirected the high-altitude experiments in which a number of victims were killed, and he was interested in continuing studies dealing with the human response to cold water and the efficacy of various rewarming techniques. Since Rascher was not considered a trained scientist, he had to collaborate with Holzloehner and Finke,[7,11,14] both of whom were scientists and were familar with this area of research. Although this research was done under the auspices of the German *SS*, the German Air Force (Luftwaffe) was also involved— even though this point was denied by Goring, head of the German Air Force, at the Nuremberg trials.[15]

Two sets of experiments were designed and implemented. The first set was one in which the human response to freezing water was determined and another set in which various rewarming techniques were evaluated. Most of the immersion hypthermia and rewarming experiments were conducted at Dachau along with some initial cold-air studies. Also, Rascher did some cold-air experiments at Auschwitz, since the air temperature was colder there than at Dachau. He was solely responsible for this cold-air phase of the experiments since Holzloehner and Finke reportedly no longer collaborated with him. The experiments that he did without the collaboration of other scientists have been shown to be fraudulent.[10,16]

The number of victims involved in the cold-water experiments is not clear, although the Alexander report claims that 130 experiments were performed. A technician of Rascher, Neff, claims 280–300 subjects were involved. Neff asserted that between 80 and 90 victims died.[17] Because Neff assisted Rascher in these experiments, his testimony was suspect. Therefore, the actual number of deaths will never be known. It has been documented that anesthetized and conscious nonconsenting prisoners of war survived a number of experiments and others did not. The following measurements were taken on these victims: internal and external temperatures, heart sounds, electrocardiograms, and chemical analysis of blood, cerebrospinal fluid, and urine.

Results

Overall, the information[17]

> documented the general physiological signs that occur with immersion hypothermia in humans and identified the cause of death from hypothermia as cardiovascular in origin, probably ventricular fibrillation. In addition the data established that rapid rewarming was effective in these subjects; that the neck and back of the head (occiput) had to be protected to minimize the effects of hypothermia; a significant increase in blood sugar and blood viscosity and that was associated with immersion hypothermia

One of the consequences of this information was the redesign of hypothermia-protective devices in which the head and neck were protected.[18]

Validity of the Data

Although Rascher was not considered a trained scientist, the presence of Holzloehner and Finke established the scientific credibility of the team. The report submitted to Himmler listed Holzloehner as the main author,[12] indicating that Holzloehner had a significant role in the experiments. Rascher might have been the instigator behind the experiments, however, he was aided by some very well trained scientists. The information from these experiments was presented at different times to the Luftwaffe and Wehrmact doctors by Holzloehner.[19,20] After the war, Holzloehner commited suicide, and Finke disappeared. Andrew Ivy, a physiologist from the University of Chicago, was the American scientist who evaluated the data for the Nuremburg trials. In his introduction to *Doctors of Infamy*, Ivy states the following:

> "Were the criminal medical experiments carried out in Nazi Germany of any real scientific value? As a matter of fact, they were not." He then goes on to say, "So the greatest of all medical tragedies was further magnified by the fact that the experiments performed added nothing of significance to medical knowledge."[16]

However, in 1947, Ivy states "that some of the data were obviously good."[21] In 1954, Ivy wrote to J. Nestor, a pediatric cardiologist in the US, that the Nazi studies had "some very worthwhile results" in that he felt the Nazis had studied, quite carefully, the effect of cooling on human beings. As he wrote to Nestor, "I had hoped at the time to collect all the worthwhile results and have them published."[22]

Ivy's turnabout on this issue is interesting, but more importantly he did consider the data accurate. He attempted to compile and publish the data. Ivy was the only scientist at that time to evaluate the data, and it is erroneously acknowledged that he did not think the data were valid.

Referencing the Data

The information from the hypothermia experiments had bearing in two areas of research: one dealing with hypothermia effects on the entire body and the other with hypothermia use in open-heart surgery. In the case of temperature regulation, there were no data available at that time that documented human response to cold water. In the case of open heart surgery, there was no safe and practical heart-lung machine in the 1950s, and surgeons were investigating ways to prolong the life of the heart by using hypothermia. The data were referenced in studies of temperature regulation[10,17,23–30] as well as in studies of the cardiovascular system.[23,24,28,31–34] This list is not complete but is presented to demonstrate that the information gathered from the hypothermia experiments designed and implemented in the concentration camps was referenced by scientists who were knowledgable in this area.

Scientific Arguments
Against the Use of the Data

There have been a number of arguments raised against the quality of the science of the hypothermia data. These arguments are:

First, since the experiments cannot be repeated, the data can never be considered accurate. The counterargument is that various aspects of the information have been referenced by scientists.[17,23–26,28–35] These articles referenced the Dachau data in the traditional sense. Specifically, the Dachau data were similar to what other scientists observed in isolated events, or they presented certain observations that led to other insights. In some cases, the referenced Dachau data in the form of graphs were actually presented in the written text.

Even if the experiments had not been duplicated, that does not disprove their accuracy. Duplication of experiments is not done in all fields of science. For example, case histories in medicine are isolated examples of some phenomenon that cannot be duplicated but are presented for discussion and to act as an impetus for studies in that area. Thus, the Dachau data could be referenced just as a case history that gave insight into a certain area of science.

Second, a number of questions have been raised concerning the methodology of the experiments, such as number of subjects, the statistical methods, the use of controls, and so forth. However, the analysis and presentation of the data were consistent with current scientific practices. One cannot evaluate scientific methodology of 50 years ago using current scientific practices. However, the scientists at Dachau were aware of scientific principles and thus cannot be considered mere novices in the area of science.

Scientific Conclusions

Overall, the following conclusions may be made:

1. There was a rationale for the experiments;
2. The experiments were conducted by trained scientists who had experience in the area of science and temperature regulation;
3. The data were presented to various scientific audiences in Nazi Germany;

4. The information has been referenced by scientists since World War II who are knowledgeable in this area; and
5. No one has scientiflcally debunked the major findings.

Concern regarding the ethical and scientific aspects of these experiments surfaced at the Nuremburg trials.[13,19,36] In addition, Alexander, Ivy, and Beecher[12,16,36] also expressed some concern as to the ethics of the experiments, and Beecher raised questions on whether this kind of data should be published or referenced.[19] Since then, there has been limited attention focused on this issue.[37]

Ethical Considerations of Referencing the Information

The use of the concentration camp data has scientific and social consequences. I have considered the data from a scientific point. What remains to be discussed are the main objections that have been raised concerning the ethical aspects of the data collection and their subsequent use. The arguments are as follows.

The methods that were used were unethical since human subjects were killed for the generation of the data. Consequently, the data are "tainted" and cannot be used. Various general statements have been made concerning this conclusion. Keeping in mind that general statements give little guidance into this problem, they are nevertheless presented for the sake of completeness. The point is made that nothing good can come from something that is evil and that the data are evil or tainted. The counterargument is that it would be best to get some good from the evil experiments and this could be accomplished by using the data to advance humankind's understanding. It is argued that in this way, the victims would not have died in vain.

Specifically, the information could theoretically be used to advance the understanding of temperature regulation and open-heart surgery either directly or indirectly and thus could help save human lives. The most powerful argument in defense of the use of the data gathered by unethical methods is that the information gathered is independent of the ethics of the methods and that the two are not linked together. In essence, data are neither evil or good.

An example that has been used to demonstrate the complexity of this position is as follows: A drug dealer whose profession has resulted in the death of individuals, the breakup of families, and the dehumanization of individuals gives a large sum of money to a local charity for the expressed purpose of helping the poor and feeding the homeless. Should the charity accept the money knowing full well the source of those funds? In essence, the question is whether or not the money is tainted. Some would argue that it would be better to feed the homeless even though the source of the funds was unethical. Others would say that it would be better not to accept the money since it is tainted and no matter how great the good it could produce, its evil genesis would always outweigh any potential benefits.

Second, if one references this data, it will acknowledge the Nazi regime and their philosophy and also encourage and support, indirectly, other unethical physician–scientists to enact similar studies. However, scientists use data gathered from a number of countries in which there is an abuse of human rights. This information is considered valid—even though it comes from a totalitarian regime. As to the second part of the objection, regretfully, there is no safeguard against a scientist–physician in a totalitarian regime conducting unethical experiments.

Another argument is that although the information has been corroborated by other scientists, the scientists who did the research were unethical and therefore, the information should be discarded. Rascher was a very unethical person in terms of torturing prisoners and so on, and therefore, anything that he did was open to suspicion and doubt. In fact, Himmler stated that he needed to have unethical scientists doing these experiments.[18] Referencing the data would send a social message that the character of a scientist is not that important. Also, referencing the data would give a sense of immortality to unethical scholars. Once an article is referenced, the authors of the work are then acknowledged by their peers as contributing to that area of science. In essence, their work continues to engender further discussions and experiments. Thus, Rascher, who was a murderer, would be acknowledged for his insights into temperature regulation. The counterargument is that there is no relationship between the ethics of an investigator and the validity of their data. A consequence of such a philosophy, in which the ethics of the investigator plays a role in determining the validity of the investigator's data, would be to have some form of "character" analysis of each scientist before/after his or her experiments. Obviously, such a scenario would undermine the freedom of scientific inquiry.

In addition, another consequence of the use of this data is that unethical scientific experiments in which human subjects are killed casts a pallor over scientific inquiry in general as well as the specific area (hypothermia). The counterargument is that the referencing of the data does not denegrate the entire area of scientific inquiry. Scientific inquiry is constantly being funded and supported, and there has been no decrease in proper, ethically conducted research.

Referencing the data condones selective dehumanization and death of those segments of society that are considered at the time "undesirable" or "expendable." The counterargument is that the referencing of the data does not condone racism or genocide. For example, the fact that a scientist uses data from a penal colony does not mean he supports the imprisonment of criminals.

The use of the information states that the collection of information is of greater value than the individuals from whom the data was gathered. The counterargument is that one has to be practical in viewing these data. It is one of a kind, cannot be reproduced, and advances humankind's understanding of certain phenomenon.

Using the data places a greater degree of importance on scientific inquiry than on ethics and consequently, could lead to a utilitarian society that would lead to a debasing of humankind. Scientific inquiry is by nature analytical and detached and has as its main goal the advancement of humankind's understanding. Ethics is the counterbalance to the thrust of scientific inquiry. It considers the long-term effects of scientific inquiry and protects, in some ways, the nature of humankind. For this reason, ethics is equally as important as scientific inquiry. Although the Dachau data are not tainted, their use would acknowledge scientific inquiry as being more important than ethics. The counterargument is that ethics is always changing and that one cannot have any universal truths in ethics that apply. The age-old saying *Do unto others as you would have them do unto you* is generally acknowledged by all cultures and enjoys widespread support. Based on this ethical standard, one would not torture or kill victims to obtain data.

Personal Reflections

In reviewing the Dachau experiments, I have come to the conclusion that the question of whether to reference the data is not easily answered. Each individual will make a personal decision regarding this issue. If a person wishes to consider the Dachau data purely from a scientific point of view, then the answer might seem quite straightforward. If the data are accurate, it would be scientifically appropriate to reference them. If one wants to consider the ethical implication of the use of these data then the decision to reference the data is not as easy. When all is said and done, it must be remembered that in these experiments, selected groups of people were slowly killed—murdered to gain scientific information. Citation of unethical data acknowledges the dehumanization and death that occurred in gathering the information and also demeans scientific inquiry. The argument that the information could be used to save human lives is a powerful one, but referencing unethical data supports the unethical implementation of experiments that might lead to more lives being lost—for the sake of gathering information—in another crisis situation. Even though the argument has been made that human subjects "had" to be used during this crisis situation, the same information could have been gathered by ethical means even during the war. In this case, the ethical considerations of the Dachau data gathered do not warrant them continuing to be scientifically referenced.

The practical question arises as to whether the unethically gathered Dachau data should be studied. This is a very difficult question. During this entire chapter, the discussion has focused on the referencing of the Dachau data. The evaluation of unpublished proceedings of inhuman experiments may lead to new insights into scientific questions that can be used to advance humankind. This endeavor does not debase humankind. To reference these experiments, however, would be acknowledging the value of scientific inquiry over ethical standards. Therefore, these data should be made available to interested scientists so that they might advance humankind's understanding. However, the source of their insight or the authors of the unethical experiments should not be acknowledged in the scientific literature.

There are some other considerations concerning the unethical Dachau experiments that need to be addressed. It is my impression that physicians as a group have been castigated because of these experiments. It should be emphasized that it was not just the medical community that participated in the design and implementation of unethical experiments in Nazi Germany but various components of the entire scientific community. Those physicians who were scientists were but part of a larger social movement. Physicians alone did not go amok; certain aspects of the entire scientific community did. It should be remembered that some members of the scientific community protested against these experiments.

Furthermore, it seems that these experiments cast a pallor on the whole area of human experimentation. Continued ethical research efforts using human subjects is paramount if we wish to advance medical science. This research should continue and not be damned because of the unethical experiments done in Nazi Germany.

The need for maintaining an integration between ethics and scientific inquiry is critical for the well being of a society that promotes individual rights. As difficult as it is, this integration must be enhanced and developed. This approach will promote the development of an ethical scientific base of knowledge that will advance the well being of humankind rather than debase it.

Acknowledgments

I would like to thank the following individuals for their assistance and guidance as I wrote this article: the staff, especially M. Pozos and C. von Rabeneau, of the Hypothermia Laboratory at University of Minnesota, Duluth, School of Medicine; and A. R. Jonsen, N. S. Jecker, and K. B. Benson of the Medical History and Ethics Department at the University of Washington School of Medicine. The patience, support, and advice of my wife, A. Pozos, is gratefully appreciated as this idea and paper evolved.

Special thanks is extended to the various ex-prisoners of Nazi concentratration camps that communicated to me their thoughts on this issue. I will fondly remember our discussions.

Nazi Science

Comments on the Validation
of the Dachau Human Hypothermia Experiments

Robert L. Berger

"It is our deep obligation to all peoples of the world to show why and how these things happened. It is incumbent upon us to set forth with conspicuous clarity the ideas and motives which moved these defendants to treat their fellow men as less than beasts. The perverse thoughts and distorted concepts which brought about these savageries are not dead. They cannot be killed by force of arms. They must not become a spreading cancer in the breast of humanity. They must be cut out and exposed, for the reason so well stated by Mr. Justice Jackson in this courtroom a year ago—'The wrongs...have been so calculated, so malignant, and so devastating, that civilization cannot tolerate their being ignored because it cannot survive their being repeated.' "[1]

Between August, 1942 and May, 1943 male prisoners of the Dachau concentration camp were forced into an ice-water bath as part of a medical research protocol on hypothermia. The victims were held in the freezing water for periods lasting as long as seven hours. Pain from contact with ice-cold water is excruciating and must have lasted until consciousness was lost. Postwar testimony disclosed that

300 men were cooled during 400 experiments indicating that many subjects were used more than once. Approximately 90 victims died during the experiments. One witness knew of only two of these men who survived the war and testified that both finished as "mental cases."[2] The German physician-investigators maintained that the project was designed to find an effective treatment for Air Force (Luftwaffe) crews downed into the cold waters of the North Sea and to save them from death through hypothermia. The doctors also claimed that their objective was accomplished.[3,4]

Full reconstruction of the concentration camp human studies has not been possible since most of the original experimental records were destroyed by the Germans before the camps were captured by the Allied Forces. Considerable information was retrieved, however, from the extensive correspondence between the investigators and Heinrich Himmler, the Nazi official who was in charge of these projects. With regard to the Dachau hypothermia experiments, Leo Alexander, a US Army psychiatrist and subsequent adviser to the Chief of Counsel for War Crimes, conducted an investigation during the immediate postwar period. He prepared a 228-page report that included, among other documents, a 68-page commentary about the background and substance of the experiments and a reproduction of a 56-page original scientific report submitted by the Dachau doctors to Himmler.[4] The latter document will be referred to in this chapter as the Dachau Scientific Report or DSR. The Alexander report has been the main source of information about the Dachau human hypothermia study and essentially the sole original reference cited on the subject in the medical literature.

The Dachau hypothermia project was condemned after the war by the civilized world outside Germany and the experiments have been regarded as crimes committed under the guise of medical research.[3-5] At first, Alexander believed that the study was scientifically sound, but subsequently changed his position and concluded that the results were not dependable.[4,6] Andrew Ivy, a physician, scientist, and representative of the American Medical Association at the Nuremberg War Criminal Trials, testified that the German concentration camp experiments were of no medical value.[3] During the ensuing years, however, scientists in the US and UK have referred to the Dachau study implying that the results were dependable and valuable.[7,8] Over time, a general impression has evolved that, in spite of its offensive ethics, the scientific base of the work was sound. The early postwar skepticism about the reliability of the data, however, re-surfaced sporadically.[8-10] Because of the lingering doubts about the scientific integrity of the project and lack of a published in-depth analysis, I embarked on a thorough examination of the background and scientific rigor of the Dachau hypothermia study. The results of the analysis were published elsewhere.[11] Highlights of the findings are summarized below.

1. The experimental approach was disorganized and haphazard. The work did not follow an orderly protocol essential for an acceptable scientific inquiry.
2. Methods of the study were inhumane and did not meet the scientific standards prevalent at the time the work was performed.
3. Conduct of the experiments was erratic and sloppy.
4. The reporting on the work was incomplete and the reported data are riddled with internal contradictions.
5. There is evidence of data falsification and suggestion of fabrication.
6. The investigators were either not familiar with or disregarded fundamental clinical and physiologic principles essential for both a sound scientific inquiry and correct interpretation of the results.
7. Many conclusions are not supported by the data presented.
8. Dr. Sigmund Rascher, the principal investigator, lacked appropriate training in investigative work and was not qualified to carry out medical research. Several of his other research efforts were judged fraudulent and were discredited.
9. Two presumably experienced collaborators, Drs. Holzloehner and Finke, were recruited to provide the expertise required for the hypothermia study, but they either did not have the authority or failed to challenge Rascher in order to ensure

   acceptable scientific standards. Both withdrew two months
   after initiation of the project. The majority of the experiments
   were performed by Rascher alone. Thus, responsibility for the
   final product rests with the unqualified Rascher.
10. Rascher's credibility is severely compromised by a consistent
    pattern of fraud and deception in his other scientific efforts
    and in his personal affairs. His integrity was eventually
    questioned even by his Nazi mentors. He was arrested in 1944
    and charged with a variety of crimes, including scientific
    fraud. Approximately one year after his imprisonment,
    Rascher was executed, presumably on Himmler's orders.
11. Heinrich Himmler, Commander of the SS, was not trained
    in medicine, yet he controlled some of the scientific aspects
    of the project.
12. The principal investigator was not trustworthy and the
    scientific process behind the experiments was deeply
    compromised. The data were not reliable and therefore their
    use cannot advance present-day research, improve on
    available therapy, or save lives.

   The Dachau study was performed almost 50 years ago,
and therefore, I exercised utmost care throughout the above
analysis to measure the work by standards prevalent at the
time the research was conducted and to avoid judgment
on a contemporary scale. It is relevant to note, however, that
in spite of the enormous progress achieved in medical science during the second half of this century, fundamental
rules of the scientific process and codes of ethics remain
largely unchanged.

   The documents retrieved from Himmler's hidden files
indicate that the DSR was prepared by Rascher for presentation at a military medical conference in Nuremberg in
1942.[12] The report is scientifically oriented and sufficiently
detailed to permit evaluation of the quality of the work. The
conclusions drawn above regarding Rascher's work are consistent with the reservations expressed about his performance
by his German superiors and colleagues, with the poor rat-
ings of his other research efforts, and with the overwhelming evidence of dishonest conduct in his professional work
and in his private affairs.[13]

The results of the in-depth analysis of the Dachau hypothermia project was published in an internationally recognized medical journal after the usual stringent peer review process. The reviewers took no exception to the criticism of the quality of the science behind the hypothermia study. A companion editorial examined the implications of the Nazi hypothermia experiments on present day unethical research. It accepted my grave misgivings about the scientific integrity of the Dachau experiments without qualification.[14] The article elicited scores of letters to the editor. Some supported the ethical stands taken in the article, many questioned the wisdom of writing the paper and criticized the journal for publishing it, but none challenged the conclusion that flawed science was practiced in Dachau. Additionally, in a published report, authored by seventeen physicians, the Committee on Bioethical Issues of the Medical Society of the State of New York concurred with my assessment of the quality of science behind the Dachua hypothermia experiment and stated that "The discussion about the possible benefits to mankind from Nazi research data should finally come to an end with the recent demonstration by Berger that the Dachau hypothermia experiments were severely flawed and yielded no scientifically valid data."[15] In the *Minnesota Daily,* Dolores Lutz reported that "After reading Berger's report Pozos told The Associated Press that the experimenters' scientific methods were 'atrocious'."[16]

The consensus in the scientific community about the unacceptable science behind the Dachau hypothermia experiments was challenged by at least two dissenting opinions, both claiming that the study offers usable scientific information. Robert Pozos, who previously called the science behind the Dachau experiments "atrocious" reverted to his original position of support for the validity of the Dachau data. In a manuscript coauthored with J. Katz, Pozos maintains that the reservations expressed in my paper have merit only if applied to the Dachau experiments "as a whole."[17] They also insist that isolated findings from the Dachau study either confirmed prior experimental data or produced new information that scientists have considered valid and therefore selected items from the Dachau experiment are reliable. It seems that in their opinion, neither the unreliability of the project "as a whole" nor the total lack of credibility of the principal investigator detracts from the integrity of the component parts. Pozos and Katz elaborate on five isolated items from the Dachau study. They attempt to prove that this subset of information is sound by using what are in my view less than convincing arguments, an inaccurate presentation of facts, and misleading or out-of-context quotations from my paper. Finally, they suggest that my unfavorable conclusions could be motivated by a desire to find evidence for rejecting the validity of Nazi studies.

The second expression of confidence in the reliability of the Dachau study came from Golden during a television presentation.[18] Like Pozos and Katz, Golden admits that the experiments were flawed, but attempts to salvage individual items for respectability and for use. In this process, the contents of the Dachau report are misinterpreted and the study is credited with having produced results that in fact it did not produce. Golden attributes the direction of his ongoing research effort on resuscitation from hypothermia to data drawn from the Dachau experiments. Ironically, there does not seem to be any connection between the work pursued by Golden and the information reported from the Dachau hypothermia project.

The current controversy over the use of the results from the Dachau hypothermia study was initiated by Robert Pozos who turned to the bioethical community as well as to the print and broadcast media to air the issue.[19-25] The dialog culminated in his endorsement of the scientific validity of the Dachau project in a recorded lecture, delivered at the University of Minnesota Symposium on the Meaning of the Holocaust for Bioethics in May, 1989.[7] In this lecture, Pozos discussed the background of the Dachau hypothermia experiments, enumerated specific items of presumably useful information generated by the study, listed the benefits already derived from using the Dachau data, projected areas of possible applications in the future, and stated that, with rare exception, scientists regard the results from Dachau as valid and useful. This discourse by Pozos provided clearly defined material for examination of the validation process itself. The present chapter will deal with the allegations advanced in the lecture endorsing the scientific health of the Dachau study. Representative claims or statements from the discourse will be quoted and will be followed by responsive comments based on available information about the Dachau human hypothermia experiments and on present-day knowledge about hypothermia.

Issues of Scientific Concern

Claim: "Golden...wrote...'It has been suggested that the experimental subjects used were likely to be emaciated and, therefore, not representative of the population as a whole. However, Alexander's report states that a variety of body types was used and specifically describes the effect of cooling on some emaciated subjects, page 49."

Comment: Alexander merely noted briefly on page 49 of his report that "emaciated people and youthful vaso-labile individuals lost their warmth more rapidly than others" without further comments or data on the body types or nutritional states of the victims.[4] There is not even a hint by Alexander that the experimental subjects were representative of the general population.

Claim: "The experiments consisted of having the subject immerse in the cold water until their core temperature had fallen to 30°C."

Comment: There is no indication in the DSR that cessation of active cooling was guided by a predetermined specific temperature level. On the contrary, the DSR reveals that neither the 30°C quoted in the above claim nor any other designated end point of cooling was incorporated into the experimental protocol. The lack of a planned systematic approach to cooling constitutes a serious defect in experimental design since each of the several end point alternatives (body temperature level, immersion time, clinical state, death, and so forth) produces a distinctly different response.

Claim: "The investigators reported some atrial fibrillation which remained even after the body warmed and this would stop spontaneously sometime after rewarming."

Comment: In fact, the term atrial fibrillation is not mentioned in the DSR. Recognition of this particular form of disturbance in cardiac rhythm would have been important since atrial fibrillation is frequently associated with hypothermia. Failure to detect this easily identifiable arrhythmia reflects a lack of expertise in ECG interpretation. This suspicion is heightened by the use in the DSR of simplistic terms instead of the universally employed specific nomenclature for characterization of cardiac rhythms. Atrial flutter, a standard designation, is mentioned once, but in that instance the companion figure in the DSR depicts a tracing of atrial fibrillation. The misinterpretation of a common ECG pattern may be another manifestation of the lack of competence in reading ECGs. In fairness, in a separate short report from Rascher to Himmler, the term atrial fibrillation is mentioned once.[26]

Claim: "The rate of cooling was five to six degrees per hour."

Comment: This cooling rate is consistent with the temperature drop and duration of cooling reported in the DSR. However, Alexander noted that examination of Rascher's experimental records and statements by his close associates revealed that the duration of immersion in fatal experiments ranged from 80 minutes to seven hours rather than the 53–100 minutes reported in the DSR. Alexander also commented that at the time the Dachau experiments were performed, it was known that the German Air Force fliers succumbed to hypothermia within 60–100 minutes of ditching into the North Sea. Rascher was determined to reproduce this time frame, regardless of the actual observations in his experiments, in order to preserve relevance of the project to the plight of the Air Force personnel.[6] Thus, it is apparent that the cooling rate cited in the validation exercise was derived from fraudulent data.

Claim: "...the body temperature continued to fall after the removal from the cold water...This phenomenon, which is called 'after drop' always occurs."

Comment: Although the claim is consistent with the information provided in the text of the DSR, the temperature curves in the same document contradict the information in the text and depict the event as a variable phenomenon. Thus, the claim that an "after drop" always occurs seems an inaccurate representation of the Dachau data and conceals one of the many internal contradictions in the reporting by the Nazi doctors.

Claim: "They established (for the first time) that the neck and the back of the head, the occiput, had to be protected to minimize the effects of hypothermia."

Comment: This claim is consistent with the information in the DSR, maintaining that inclusion of the neck and occiput into the ice bath greatly accelerated cooling and that death or cerebral hemorrhage was limited to victims with the more inclusive immersion. The latter assertion from Dachau also implies that immersion in cold water is unlikely to result in death unless the neck and occiput are included in the coolant liquid and suggests that a fatal outcome can be prevented by keeping these structures out of the water. Although it is known that the scalp is an efficient heat-exchanging surface, the lethal influence assigned to cooling of the neck and head by the Dachau researchers has not been confirmed by extensive experience with hypothermia during the last 45 years.[27,28] The concept of the importance of local cooling of the neck and occiput was promulgated by Himmler. Gagge and Harrington commented in a review of the Dachau project that "...it cannot be said that any convincing explanation of the extraordinary quantitative effect of the local cooling of the neck and occiput is available. It is probable that the effect is qualitatively real, and conceivable that the disparity was quantitatively exaggerated for the benefit of H. Himmler."[9]

Claim: "They did show that alcohol was not effective in terms of increasing the rate of hypothermia nor was it effective in terms of rewarming."

Comment: In fact, the DSR informs that pretreatment with alcohol accelerates both cooling and rewarming. Furthermore, Harold Laufman noted that the influence of alcohol in the Dachau study could not be evaluated since "...the amount given was very small and the posthypothermic observations were inadequate."[10]

Claim: "They established (for the first time) that rapid rewarming was effective."

Comment: The term rapid rewarming refers to treatment by immersion in a warm water bath. The most important criterion for the effectiveness of a rewarming technique is survival. Since the DSR fails to furnish survival statistics, how can one judge the effectiveness of rapid or any other rewarming therapy? The validity of the claim about the superiority of warm bath resuscitation in the Dachau setting is further compromised by testimony of an assistant who revealed that some victims were thrown into boiling water for rewarming and most of them died.[29] It is doubtful that the use of a technique with substantial inherent lethal threat influenced survival rates favorably. Thus, contrary to the claim by the validator, the effectiveness of rapid rewarming was not demonstrated by the Dachau study. Actually, its role in resuscitation from hypothermia remains controversial even to this day.[30]

Claim: "Death usually occurred somewhere between 24 and 25°C."

Comment: This claim refers to the lethal temperature levels reported in the text of the DSR. However, a companion table in the same document contradicts the data in the text and maintains that the victims died between 25.7 and 29.2°C. To continue the inconsistency, Rascher noted in a short intermediate report that all victims died upon reaching 28°C,[26] whereas a postscript to the DSR maintains that with a few exceptions, the lethal temperature was 26–27°C. Postwar testimony indicates that the temperature was usually lowered to 25°C.[5] Moreover, the lethal temperatures are provided only from a small population and no information is supplied about the final level of hypothermia in the large majority of experimental deaths. In addition, the mortality rate at the critical temperature level is not specified, which means that the lethality of the "lethal" temperature is not available. Thus, the endorser presented only selected as well as incomplete information from the DSR on the lethal limits of hypothermia and failed to call attention to the inconsistencies in the data. Through this approach, the unreliability of the results reported from Dachau seems to have been concealed.

Claim: "According to Dr. Holzloehner death always was due to ventricular fibrillation. Overall, the Dachau data used (sic) on these non-consenting prisoners of war showed for the first time the following:...and that more than likely the cause of death was ventricular fibrillation."

Comment: The term ventricular fibrillation does not appear in the DSR. Death is attributed to heart failure from structural myocardial damage and other contributing factors that suggest a mechanism distinctly different from primary ventricular fibrillation. Although Alexander mentioned in his report that he was informed after the war that Holzloehner attributed death to ventricular fibrillation, this impression is not supported by the DSR. Moreover, without ECG monitoring during critical phases of the experiments and with the investigators' dubious expertise in ECG interpretation, ventricular fibrillation could not have been identified as the cause of death in Dachau.

Claim: "Is there still some data that might be relevant to modern day studies on hypothermia? Yes, there are. The German scientists reported that there was an increase in cerebral edema in hypothermic victims."

Comment: Contrary to the results reported from Dachau, it has been established that the levels of hypothermia reached in these experiments protect the brain instead of damaging it. As a matter of fact, various degrees of subnormal temperatures are employed for preservation of tissue viability in a wide variety of clinical situations. For example, in order to protect the brain and the rest of the body, hypothermia is routinely induced during 250,000–300,000 heart operations peformed annually, in the US alone, without concern about cerebral edema from lowering the body temperature. The cerebral edema reported from Dachau was either pure fabrication or may have been produced by causes other than hypothermia, i.e., from shock or brain injury due to beating or to struggle during cooling. Considering the known absence of a causal relationship between the levels of hypothermia reached at Dachau and cerebral edema, it is curious that the alleged connection is represented as credible observation and as "relevant to modern day studies on hypothermia."

Claim: "The data was (sic) presented at scientific meetings in Germany and nowhere has (sic) it (sic) been...questioned."

Comment: In fact, after presentation of the Dachau study at a Nuremberg military medicine conference in 1942, Grosse Buckhoff, a prominent physiologist, questioned the need or justification for human studies and noted that the data did not add materially to the knowledge obtained through animal experimentation.[31] It may also be relevant that a book on the achievements of German aviation medicine during World War II, written by German scientists, devoted a lengthy discussion to hypothermia, but failed to mention Rascher's name or his work.[32]

Issues of Concern About Claims on the Background and Implications of the Study

The discussion in the lecture of endorsement presented by Pozos at the Symposium on the Meaning of the Holocaust for Bioethics was not limited to the scientific arena. It also included issues about the background and implications of the study. Concern was professed about the brutality of the Dachau project yet, in my view, obvious bias was exhibited in favor of the experimentors coupled with derogatory insinuations about the character of the victims. The lecturer implied that the experiments were necessary, justified, and not as inhumane as commonly perceived. The endorser referred to specific clinical benefits obtained from using the Dachau data when in fact these attributions are without foundation. Critics of the experiments were discredited and supporters were embraced. The following examples will illustrate the point.

Statement: " To a large extent the mastery of these kinds of questions as well as others, were (sic) essential for the survival of a nation engaged in a war effort."

Comment: The statement echoes the pronouncements by Himmler and the Nazi propaganda. It distorts reality and justifies the entire Dachau effort by maintaining that the experiments were necessary. Can survival of a nation justify or hinge on inhumane pseudoscientific experiments by a man known for fraudulent and incompetent medical research?

Statement: "Were these experiments necessary...could the Germans have received the data another way...was this really something they had to do, or was it an excuse?...there was no data out there that they could turn to."

Comment: Not even the unavailability of the desired data justifies the inhumanity of the Dachau experiments. Moreover, at least one prominent World War II German physiologist, Grosse-Buckhoff, felt that the information obtained from the human project was already available from animal studies.[31]

Statement: "Regretfully the idea of using prisoners who were condemned to die is a very old tradition...the Germans were continuing a long, gory history...They are not the first and I do not believe that they will be the last."

Comment: Most concentration camp inmates were not sentenced to death by a legal process. Moreover, the gross inhumanity of the Dachau experiments had not been traditional, but rather unprecedented in the history of medical research. Thus, the analogy is inaccurate. Lastly, even a long history of inhumane practice fails to justify continuation of the unacceptable.

Statement: "Is this situation so unique that there is no counterpart in history and that these experiments require special admonition? All experiments that have used nonconsenting subjects should be admonished....But what is interesting to me is that the Japanese in World War II, under the command of another physiologist, Dr. Ishi, conducted experiments on human subjects...Hubert (an American official) agreed to take the Japanese, to give them immunity in return for their cooperation. Dr. Ishi, five years ago, was awarded the Outstanding Award in Japan for his work on temperature regulation in humans."

Comment: Is this an attempt to condone one evil by citing another?

Statement: "This attorney then goes on to state that many of the physicians who were involved in these experiments had to do these experiments because they were forced to do them at a point of a gun. He, the attorney, had great sympathy for the 'victims of Nuremberg' as he called them...there were a number of physicians who did not take part in the experiments.

Comment: The notion that the German physicians were reluctant participants in the Nazi brutalities and complied only "at a point of a gun" is inaccurate. We know that the German medical profession played a major role in the formulation and implementation of Hitler's racial agenda. German doctors embraced the Nazi program and participated even in its most brutal practices voluntarily and usually with enthusiasm. There were a few German physicians in the concentration camps who declined to accept specific assignments they found objectionable and were not penalized.[33] Lastly, giving credence to a man who had "great sympathy" for the Nazi doctors, convicted of crimes against humanity, and who refers to mass murderers as "the Nuremberg victims," cannot be viewed as objective or without prejudice.

Claim: "...the credibility of the data is considered to be in question because of the training of Rascher...the presence of Holzloehner and Finke established the credibility of the team."

Comment: Available documents indicate that Holzloehner and Finke participated essentially as part-time consultants and did not direct the hypothermia experiments at Dachau. They withdrew even from a limited collaboration after approximately 50 of the 400 experiments had been completed. There is convincing evidence that the project was controlled by Rascher and the experiments were performed under his supervision.[5,34] Thus, transfer of responsibility for quality control from the unqualified Rascher to the presumably more competent Holzloehner and Finke, in an attempt to salvage credibility, cannot be justified from available description on the organizational structure of the project.

Claim: "A personal account that had been told by one of the survivors of the hypothermia experiments was that the subjects that were chosen for these experiments were chosen by the prisoners and that in many cases the ones that were chosen were those who had a criminal record or were creating problems in the barracks."

Comment: Available information indicates that the victims were selected by the political section of the SS and the choice had to be approved by the camp commandant.[34] This approach is more consistent with our knowledge of concentration camp practices than with the policy suggested by the endorser's account.[35] The claim also implies that the victims were not innocent men but undesirable elements who deserved punishment.

Claim: "In talking to some of these people who were involved in these hypothermic experiments, the screaming was more than likely staged, because when you are becoming hypothermic, ladies and gentlemen, there is no way you are going to scream. The most you are going to be able to do is to impair your respiration and finally you become hypothermic and lose the ability to articulate at all. More than likely what was happening...they were smart, and what they were doing was staging that they were having extreme difficulty so that Neff (Rascher's assistant) supposedly could stop the experiments."

Comment: Once hypothermia destroys the ability to phonate, neither staged nor spontaneous screaming is possible. Thus, the attempt to create a connection between staged screaming and the hypothermic state lacks both logic and physiological basis. The claim also implies that the victims

were schemers, whereas the experimentors were compassionate men who would be moved by the suffering of the freezing
prisoners and halt the torture. In fact, the victims did not
have to fake misery. Immersion in ice-cold water is bitterly
painful. The screaming from the ice tank must have come
during the early stages of cooling when speech was still intact.
It must have been a spontaneous response to the pain of
freezing. The noise was so loud and terrifying that it proved
upsetting even in a concentration camp. It did not elicit sympathy or reprieve. Rascher simply requested relocation of the
project to the larger Auschwitz facility where the experiments
could be sequestered to a remote site and the screaming would
be kept away from the earshot of the main camp.

Claim: "However in a letter sent to Dr. Nestor, a cardiovascular surgeon... Dr. Ivy basically in that letter contradicts
what he wrote in the *Doctors of Infamy*. Dr. Ivy is the only
scientist who has ever contradicted the data. Dr. Ivy's background has nothing to do with temperature regulation. He
was a physiologist, a full professor, whose interest was gas-
trointestinal physiology and hormone physiology...The
point I want to emphasize here, ladies and gentlemen, is I
think, for the first time I have documentation that Ivy contradicted himself and he is the only person, as I've said, who
is a physiologist who looked at the data who said it wasn't
anything worthwhile."

Comment: Regardless of the merits of the reservations
expressed about Ivy, it is relevant to note that it does not
require a hypothermia specialist to evaluate the scientific
process behind a hypothermia research effort. Furthermore,
scientists other than Ivy questioned the reliability of the
Dachau report. The list includes Leo Alexander, A. P. Gagge,
E. Harrington, and Harold Laufman. In addition, John
Hayward noted that even though the temperature levels are
not reliable, the shapes of some cooling curves are useful,
but he "wouldn't trust any of the other information."[8] Harnett
cited the Nazi data, but "admits that they are weak...uses
them only to corroborate more reliable experimental results..."[8]

Statement: "...although Rascher was killed, more than likely for producing fraudulent data, the data in the area of hypothermia stands (sic) the test for being corroborated by outside investigators....Dr. Ivy himself fell into scientific disrepute...That (sic) data (Ivy's) was (sic) found to be fraudulent...I sometimes wonder if he didn't think that some of the work that Rascher had done earlier on his thesis had some validity."

Comment: The corroboration of Rascher's work by outside investigators is open to question. In addition, Ivy's problems and the speculation about his private thoughts have no bearing on the quality of Rascher's research effort. The attempt to connect the two unrelated issues and thereby promote the reliability of Rascher's data is bizarre.

Statement: "...Mr. Neff's testimony which was used at the Nuremberg trial had to be called into question because he himself was sort of on the hot seat and people really don't understand or believe that his testimony is that reliable."

Comment: Neff was a German assistant to Rascher and gave damaging testimony about the Dachau hypothermia experiments.[34,36] He may or may not have been totally truthful, but the substance of his description about life and death at the Dachau experimental station was corroborated by other sources.[35] Neff was regarded as a credible witness at the Nuremberg War Crime Trials.

Claim: "Was the data used for any practical application?... Dr. Nestor, a cardiovascular surgeon reported to me that the data gathered from Dachau was the basis for the beginning of doing cardiac surgery using hypothermia. He states that before he had access to these experiments, relatively little was known about how cold to get patients and how long could they survive. He acknowledges this in the Medical Annals of the District of Columbia in 1955."

Comment: Nestor was not a cardiovascular surgeon, but a pediatric cardiologist and therefore in all likelihood did not perform heart surgery.[37] His name is not associated with the development of cardiac surgery under hypothermia. It is generally acknowledged that the use of hypothermia for cardiac surgery was based on the pioneering animal research by W. G. Bigelow, who was aware of the Dachau study, but did not use the results in his work and made only cursory reference to them.[38] In 1953, Lewis reported on the successful closure of an atrial septal defect with the aid of hypothermia, but did not refer to the Dachau study.[39] In the early part of 1954, a larger clinical experience with cardiac surgery under hypothermia was reported by Swan's group but again, the article did not mention the Nazi experiments.[40] Lewis' paper appeared two years before Nestor coauthored an article on four heart operations under hypothermia.[41,42] The Dachau experiments were discussed in Nestor's publication, but it was stated that "...After the war independently and without the benefit of detailed knowledge of the wartime experiments on human beings by the Nazis, Swan, Virtue and others....developed a practical technic of direct surgery of the human heart with hypothermia. Swan's method has been used satisfactorily by others including our own group, and it is this technic that we shall describe." Thus, it is evident that the data from Dachau were not used in the development of heart surgery. It is also clear that Nestor's access to the Dachau results was of no consequence since he was not one of the developers or practitioners of hypothermic cardiac surgery. It should further be noted that in the operations described by Nestor, the Dachau results were not used, but rather the technique pioneered by Swan's group was followed, and that the contents of Nestor's paper were apparently misrepresented. Thus, crediting the Dachau study as "the basis for the beginning of doing cardiac surgery using hypothermia" seems totally inaccurate, as does the identification of Nestor as a cardiovascular surgeon.

Claim: "...could this (sic) data have been used to save persons lives at the time of the experiments or immediately after World War II if this (sic) data was (sic) known? Yes... Reading the paper titled: 'Report of a Case in which the Patient Died During Therapeutic Reduction of Body Temperature with Metabolic and Pathologic Studies,' Archives of Internal Medicine 1955, it was clear that the authors were not aware of the after drop phenomenon where the patient who got cold while out of a cold situation was going to continue to get cold. That information more than likely could have saved that patient."

Comment: The patient referred to had a 5°F temperature "after drop" following termination of therapeutic cooling. Rewarming was then instituted. He died one hour later from circulatory collapse probably secondary to massive peripheral vasodilitation during rewarming and unrelated to a temperature "after drop." The paper referred to in the *Archives of Internal Medicine* was, in fact, published in 1941 and not in 1955, as claimed in the validation effort.[43] The patient died in June 1940, more than two years before the Dachau experiments were performed and more than five years before the data became available to the American medical community.[37] Obviously, the Dachau results could not have been used to benefit the patient at the time he died.

Claim: "Is there some negative reaction to not publishing the data? ... In 1960, a Dr. Fay reported that he was going to stop doing the research on hypothermia in this country even though his data showed some promise...of minimizing the growth of cancer because of the stigma attached to hypothermia research...he would be accused of doing Dachau-like experiments."

Comment: In a 1959 publication Fay reviewed more than 20 years of personal experience with therapeutic hypothermia.[44] He was enthusiastic about his work and gave no indication of an intent to retrench because of concern about accusations of doing "Dachau-like experiments." Judging from the printed discussion of the paper, Fay's presentation was well received. No one expressed ethical reservations about Fay's work and no one compared it to the Dachau experiments. Fay mentioned that the Nazi atrocities discouraged the clinical use of hypothermia temporarily, but then he continued that an accelerated interest was manifested subsequently as the benefits of the hypothermic state were demonstrated. Indeed, clinical activity with hypothermia had increased in the 1950s. According to Sealy, in 1950, there were only 16 entries in the *Index Medicus* on the clinical applications of hypothermia, but during 1960, the number grew to almost 300.[45]

Issues of Concern

The endorsing discourse at the Symposium on the Meaning of the Holocaust for Bioethics was replete with pronouncements that speak for themselves and require little comment. The following examples illustrate:

> "...and it should be emphasized that not all the subjects who were used in these experiments died."

> "The point to be made here is that there cannot be any correlation between the ethics of a scientist and the data that he or she produces."

> "Ladies and gentlemen, there is no way you are going to stop an investigator if he or she wants to do these (Nazi-like) experiments."

> "That in this society we have acknowledged science as the religion."

> "...but the point I would like to make is the situation is one where I think good might come from evil. Besides, the information that can be used to save human lives, the data could also be used to study the social pathology of humans in these situations."

Discussion

The inhumanity of the Dachau hypothermia project surpasses the unethical and assumes blatant criminal dimensions. Its scientific integrity is so severely compromised that the results are not usable. Yet, selected data from the study have been represented as valuable, with potential for advancing contemporary hypothermia research and therapy. The phenomenon is bizarre, and one can only speculate about the paradox of the poor scientific quality of the Dachau product and the favorable reception of its results. Pre-Nazi German medical research enjoyed a reputation of excellence, and to some measure, this perception persisted in spite of the drastic changes in its orientation and quality during Hitler's reign. It may have seemed inconceivable, to some investigators, that the traditionally superb standards of German medicine could deteriorate to a point where it not only tolerated but taught and practiced torture, murder, and genocide through a brand of pseudoscience. Failure to appreciate the disintegration of the previously high caliber German medical research during the Nazi era, combined with a tendency to accept data from a usually reliable source could have been responsible for citing the Dachau experiments without paying close attention of the quality of the work. The error was probably compounded by using secondary sources in the literature instead of securing and perusing the original material. This shortcut may have been prompted by the rather difficult availability of the Alexander document. Reluctance to acknowledge that the primary material was not pursued or used could account for the inappropriate listing of the Alexander paper, instead of the secondary article, as the reference. Unfortunately, the obvious violations of human standards and the lingering doubts about the scientific integrity of the experiments did not raise sufficient concern to examine the reliability of the data more closely. To compound the problem, repeated references to the Dachau study in the medical literature by respected investigators may have reinforced the impression that the scientific base of the study was sound. This false perception was temporarily fortified by the recent attempt at direct validation of the data through the lecture at the University of Minnesota Symposium. Whatever the explanation, the citing of an obvious scientific fraud as a source of dependable information by reputable investigators is disquieting.

The lecture on validation at the Symposium on the Meaning of the Holocaust for Bioethics sent an unmistakable signal that the speaker wishes to convince that the Dachau hypothermia experiments were necessary as well as justified, and that the results are valid, with potential for advancing present-day hypothermia research and therapy. Furthermore, the presentation also incorporated a veiled attempt to counter the widely held contempt for the Nazi study by promoting the appeal and credibility of the investigators while questioning the plight and character of the victims. However, the effort to validate the Dachau project was, in my opinion, riddled with serious shortcomings. The experimental design and methods of the study were not subjected to critical analysis. The available information from Dachau appears distorted and presented in an undeservedly favorable light, creating a false impression that the scientific process had been sound. Omissions of important steps in the conduct of the experiments, essential for an acceptable scientific inquiry, were concealed by attribution to the Dachau study procedures that were not, in fact, included in the work. The abundance of conflicting, fraudulent, and incomplete data reported from Dachau was not divulged. Representation of the results struck me as inaccurate and misleading. False data seemed depicted as credible information. Claims were advanced about past benefits from the use of the Dachau results that in fact had not been realized. Nonexistent life-saving potential of the Dachau data was emphasized without offering what I viewed as concrete or reliable information that could be applied to save lives. Contents of the Alexander report and those of other articles in the medical literature were misinterpreted. Conflicts between the Dachau data and well-established physiologic concepts were not revealed. Responsibility for the scientific standards was shifted, without justification in my view, from an unqualified and dishonest investigator to competent and presumably credible scientists.

Inferior scientific products are usually discarded by scientists and questions about their use do not come to the attention of ethicists. Ethical deliberations deal mostly with issues of proven scientific merit, but questionable moral implication. The conclusive evidence about the compromised scientific base of the Dachau hypothermia experiments renders the ethical discussion about the use of the results moot, inappropriate, and even harmful. Had it been appreciated that the data from Dachau are not reliable, the entire effort would have been dismissed by scientists and the ethical debate probably never would have gotten off the ground. A recent article in the *Hastings Center Report* speaks to the point.[46] Dr. A is a hypothermia scientist who believes that the information from the Dachau human hypothermia experiments is reliable and considers it particularly important to an ongoing project. Dr. A would like to use the material and refers the dilemma about disposition of the ethically compromised, but scientifically sound data to a panel of ethicists. Had Dr. A doubted the validity of the information, he/she would have rejected the study on a scientific basis, would not have felt the need to use the data or to consult the ethicists, and the issue would not have appeared in the *Hastings Center Report*. In another hypothetical situation, ethical advice is sought about the use of a life-saving therapy discovered through experiments that employed criminal methods. Before accepting the task, would not the ethicists wish to be assured that the scientific process leading to the discovery had been sound and that the therapy under consideration indeed possessed potential for saving lives? Furthermore, if information had surfaced after commencement of the dialog that the science behind the new therapy was fraudulent or that the treatment could not save lives, the discussion about the use of the data would be undoubtedly terminated. However, the decision does not have to affect further dialog about the ethical violations perpetrated at Dachau. Similarly, with documentation that the information from the Dachau project is not reliable and therefore not usable, the discussion on the use of the results becomes inappropriate and misleading. Discontinuation of the dialog about the Dachau experiments, however, does not diminish the need to confront the general issue of Nazi human experimentation.

Nazi "science" represents a shameful, but consequential phenomenon in the history of human experimentation and is highly relevant to contemporary and future practices. It cannot be written off as an aberration by Rascher and other fringe elements, since the Nazi agenda was also embraced by mainstream scientists, including physicians with impressive credentials. Medical science in the Third Reich produced the Dachau hypothermia experiments and a disturbing array of similar pseudoscientific work, but it was also responsible for a flock of scientifically credible, though often grossly inhumane projects. The industrialized Nazi killing machine that snuffed out millions of innocent lives through gassing and incineration proved to be a highly sophisticated and efficient scientific creation. Furthermore, the sordid experiments were not conducted in a remote, barbaric, or primitive society, but by scientists of a nation in the center of western civilization with a highly developed and cultured tradition. It is difficult to understand how scientists of a people that produced Goethe, Heine, Beethoven, and Einstein could be followers of a Hitler and feeders of human gas chambers. The Nazi reign showed the dark side of the German people and flagged the evil potential of humans anywhere. Unethical and inhuman medical experiments have not been limited to Nazi Germany, but have been perpetrated from time to time in other societies. If civilization is to survive, we have to learn our lessons from the Nazi experience and identify some of the forces responsible for the conversion from the civilized to the barbarous. We must develop the wisdom and the means to prevent any repetition. Continuation of the dialog about the use of the results from Dachau, however, will not advance the cause of a safe and humane approach to medical experimentation. It will only keep alive the misconception that the unspeakable horrors perpetrated by a regime intent on destroying civilization benefited humanity—or simply that in this instance, evil brought good. The present ethical discussion about the use of the Dachau data implies that the experiments have scientic merit, it tends to exonerate the perpetrators, advances the cause of Holocaust revisionist intent of falsifying history, and lends credibility to the notion that evil and fraud in science can be beneficial for humans and humankind. Banning citation of the Dachau study, however, would not be constructive and is not the way of a free society. The Alexander Report should be disseminated as a historical document that records a facet of the Holocaust, when a nation, its science, and its scientists, went mad, and physicians replaced a time-honored obligation to serve their patients with exclusive or blind loyalty to a state and to an ideology.

From approximately 30 concentration camp human experiments on record,[47] the Dachau hypothermia project has been singled out for attention, but other concentration camp studies may be revived from time to time. It is most improbable that research performed with the relatively primitive technology and limited knowledge of the 1940s, frequently with ideologues of dubious qualification, would be usable in the contemporary world of medicine. It is imperative that any Nazi medical data or other unethically obtained information under consideration for use shoud be subjected to scientific scrutiny before embarking on an ethical dialog. In the event that the work matches or resembles the flawed standards of the Dachau effort, it will be rejected because of its scientific shortcomings and a futile, or even harmful, dialog will be thereby avoided.

From: *When Medicine Went Mad* Ed.: A. Caplan
©1992 The Humana Press Inc.

The Dachau Hypothermia Study

An Ethical and Scientific Commentary

Jay Katz and Robert S. Pozos

Robert Berger has recently published an article that reevaluates the scientific merits of the hypothermia experiments conducted by Nazi physicians at Dachau.[1] On the basis of his analysis of the available, though incompletely recovered data, he concludes that these studies are scientifically flawed and therefore must be rejected "on purely scientific grounds." At the very end of his article, Berger asserts that "[t]he Dachau study is an inappropriate example for the debate over the use of unethically obtained data."

We believe that acceptance of Berger's invitation to close debate would be wrong. The controversy over what transpired at Dachau and the use of unethically obtained data—valid or invalid—remains inextricably intertwined. These debates should not be consigned to oblivion because, in his judgment, the data are useless.

Berger's analysis, viewed from the perspective of the entire project of the hypothermia experiments conducted by the Nazi physicians, raises questions about the validity of these data if taken as a whole. Thus, if judgment on validity is based on the project as a whole, his conclusions have merit.

However, as we shall soon demonstrate, individual findings are reported that either confirmed prior experimental data or produced new data that scientists in the West have considered valid and have cited in scientific journals in support of their own research findings. Moreover, the Nazi studies were conducted in the name of science and medicine to obtain scientifically valuable data.

Thus, the Dachau studies continue to haunt us not only because of what physician-scientists attempted to accomplish then, but also because of the uses to which physician-scientists have put the data since. That Berger's analysis now may allow physician-scientists to disown what they once embraced only teaches us that the Dachau experiments remain an *appropriate* example of debating the ethical implications of the use of such data.

We emphasize this lesson because too many physicians and scientists would prefer to forget that the concentration camp experiments were conducted and subsequently cited in the name of medicine and science. Proof of the flawed scientific nature of these studies would come as a welcome relief and permit us not to confront a question of ethics that the Nazi physicians bequeathed to us: Should the data, obtained under conditions of unspeakable cruelty, be used if their validity had not been in question?

We believe that even with respect to the validity of some of the individual data obtained by the Nazi physicians the verdict is not in:

1. In the Dachau data, the Nazi scientists demonstrated that the rate of cooling of human subjects in cold water was linear or at least near-linear.[2] This finding has not been contradicted in more recent studies, except for the observation that immediately after immersion, rectal temperatures remain constant for approximately 10–15 minutes.
2. The fact that there was an afterdrop—a continued cooling of the body after it was removed from the cold water—was confirmed by the Dachau scientists.[3] Although it may be variable and its mechanism not clearly understood, the fact that there is an afterdrop has not been rejected by the scientific community.

3. While the data on a crucial aspect of the hypothermia experiments—the assessment of the temperature level at which death occurs—are not consistent[4] (and perhaps cannot be because of the many variables involved), they establish a range—24.2–29.2°C—of temperatures that will prove fatal. Obviously, these data cannot be verified in civilized experimental studies.

4. The fact that various methods of rewarming reversed hypothermia in humans was extensively investigated in, and documented by, the Dachau experiments.[5] Today it is taken for granted that hypothermia can be reversed. Although different methods of rewarming exist today, the Dachau data were among the first to establish this fact.

5. Later in his article, Berger states that "[t]he concept that local application of cold to the occiput and dorsal neck accelerates cooling was advanced by Himmler and is demonstrated *convincingly* in the Dachau Comprehensive Report with the temperature curves from one set of experiments."[6] While later in the same paragraph, Berger states that "this observation was *probably* fabricated,"[7] this finding apparently has not yet been sufficiently investigated to permit a definite conclusion one way or the other. Therefore, for now, that sentence alone may contain the essence of a valid scientific observation. If all the rest of the Dachau data were fraudulent and this one fact proves not to be, one can argue that the Dachau experiments constitute a historical model for the study of the consequences of the use of unethically derived data.

Thus, Berger's article is important, not because it closes the debate over the use of unethically obtained data, but because it raises a key question in the discussion about the use of unethically gathered valid data. The question is: Granted that not all conclusions in the Dachau experiments were substantiated, does that negate those observations that were substantiated? In other words, can scientists be selective in terms of what they wish to extract from these experiments?

The goal of science is to produce new knowledge. If, during unethically conducted experiments, one valid scientific fact is produced, should that information be used as it has been, referenced in the literature as it has been, or just discarded?

Berger's conclusions deserve further scrutiny by scientists who are experts in hypothermia research because any judgment on the invalidity of the hypothermia studies in their entirety, as well as of the many other experiments conducted by Nazi physicians at Dachau, could be affected by motivations to find evidence for rejecting their validity out of concern that if valid, the studies:

1. Would, in some eyes, rehabilitate the Nazi physicians by having to admit that they did good in the midst of evil;
2. Will further disabuse us of a long-cherished assumption, most recently advanced by Nicholas Wade in *The New York Times*, that "any experiment grossly deficient in ethics is likely to be defective in other ways as well."[8] (Marcia Angell, in her editorial accompanying the Berger article, convincingly contests this assertion[9]); and
3. Would compel their use for the sake of humankind (far better to avoid this ethical dilemma).

While we believe that some of the hypothermia data are valid, we wish to emphasize again that in addition to the controversy over validity-invalidity, there is another issue that concerns us even more deeply; even if invalid, in light of what the Nazi physicians attempted to accomplish, the following question must not be evaded: To what uses should we put the data if they turn out to be valid? It is a question that for the victims' and our sake we should confront rather than allow ourselves to be comforted by the conclusion that the hypothermia or other concentration camp experiments contributed nothing to the advancement of science. Moreover, we must do so in order not to sweep under the rug many important facts:

1. That side by side with the controversial physician-scientist Sigmund Rascher, other competent and renowned scientists participated in and supported the concentration camp research;
2. That scientists throughout the West, however uncritical of their ethical implications, have made use of the data;
3. That many scientists would now use the data if they are proven to be scientifically valid; and

4. That physician-scientists, in less egregious ways, still continue to value knowledge more than respect for research subjects.

The tensions between advancement of knowledge and respect for the subjects of research persists in today's world. As Angell reminds us "unethical research continues today."[10] However, she regards this sad fact as determined more by "thoughtlessness" than "cruelty." Yet, although it may not be cruelty, it is not only thoughtlessness that contributes to the conduct of unethical research; it is equally, or even more importantly, influenced by physician-scientists' often all too relentless dedication to the ideology of advancing science, their quest for faster and better results, and their self-interest in publishing first. Thus, the Dachau study, even if it were demonstrated that the data are invalid, remains a most instructive example for the debate over the use of unethically obtained data. Views to the contrary would have had to consider whether the focus on validity speaks only to the issue of use or seeks to avoid debate on another chapter in the history of science, medicine, and humanity during which too few questions were raised about harvesting the fruits of a poisoned tree when the fruits seemed scientifically palatable.

From: *When Medicine Went Mad* Ed.: A. Caplan
©1992 The Humana Press Inc.

Moral Analysis
and the Use of
Nazi Experimental Results

Benjamin Freedman

Are the results of Nazi experiments valid? Are generalizations from those results valuable?[1] These questions are beyond the philosopher's competence. His or her task can only begin when those issues are resolved.

A moral discussion of the use of Nazi data[2] must proceed on the presumption that at least some of those results are both valid and valuable. This is obvious in the case of one who concludes that the results may be used. It is equally true, though less obvious, in the case of one who rejects the use of the data on moral grounds, for it is only after the threshold question of value and validity has been resolved that the moral question arises. The moral stance that the data must never be used could not rest easy upon the historic happenstance that none of the results are of scientific interest.

This discussion, therefore, proceeds on the presumption that at least some data are valid and valuable. At the time I originally prepared this discussion, I did in fact believe that the hypothermia data set and generalizations satisfied these conditions. Robert Berger argued, in a paper that appeared after I had prepared the following,[3] that this is a mistake. In that paper, he conclusively demonstrates critical shortcomings of the data as judged by the norms of modern medical literature. He further argues, in ways that I find convincing but not conclusive, that the data are too flawed to support any clinical generalization or proposed therapeutic innovation.

As a philosopher, of course, my beliefs on this matter are of little more than biographical interest. The hypothetical question remains: Could valid and valuable Nazi data morally be used? Given the most liberal scientific reading of the worth of the data, the issue was never more than one on the scientific periphery. Its place on the ethical map is different. The question is of profound ethical and emotional significance.

Preliminary

Let me note at the outset two difficulties in my title, in the concept of "using" Nazi experimental results. The first ambiguity that arises concerns which results will qualify as "Nazi." Robert Pozos' discussion deals with the use of results obtained during the Nazi interregnum, largely within the walls of the concentration and death camps. These results are unequivocally within the scope of Nazi data. They will therefore be the focus of my later discussion.

William Seidelman, however, has reminded us of another set of scientific studies that may be included: the work of forerunners and founding fathers of Nazi biological ideology like Ernst Rudin and Otmar von Verschuer.[4] Their work before, during, and following the Nazi era constitute unified wholes. This work was naturally accommodated within the Nazi universe; contributed to it; and in that sense, perpetuated it thereafter. Pozos speaks of data that are the grim fruit of Nazi experience; Seidelman, of the seed from which that fruit has come.

Several arguments that are made against the use of Nazi results will encompass the seed at least as well as the fruit. If that is so, however, we are reminded that this discussion has a broader ambit than anticipated, for the work of Rudin and von Verschuer remains at the root of modern psychiatry and genetics as well as of the Nazi enterprise itself. As we consider the morality of using this data, we must resist the temptation of relying upon the fortuitous fact that the most notorious results, such as those on hypothermia, are of marginal significance to medical science and practice. It could have been otherwise; perhaps, in the case of Rudin and von Verschuer, it was otherwise. To be genuinely principled, a stance on the Nazi results would have to be robust enough to forthrightly reject data of central importance to the later progress of medicine.

What is meant, next, by "using" data?

1. Data can be referred to, by citation or otherwise, serving as a presumptive empirical substrate for a scientific argument.
2. Data can ground a medical conclusion that can then serve to establish, validate, or justify clinical practice.
3. Data can serve to suggest further areas for inquiry.

The term, "the use of data," equivocates between these three different meanings; moreover, the three meanings fail in combination to exhaust the meanings attaching to the term. Until clarification of this question is achieved, it will clearly be hard to reach an ethical conclusion about the use of the data.

The first meaning might prohibit published and unpublished citation, and might prohibit the pursuit of protocols whose scientific grounding is crucially reliant upon these results. A prohibition with respect to the second meaning, "use as grounding clinical practice," might require that use of a therapy proved superior by the data be avoided—in other words, that a known inferior technique be used on the patients. The third meaning, use as suggestive of lines of inquiry, may be both the most frequent and the most evanescent way of using data. The moral implications of its prohibition are not easily drawn: perhaps, consciously induced amnesia.

These two clarifications are more than a debater's tactic. Some writers argue against "use" of the Nazi results, but are also against censoring such use. These stances are consistent if the rejection of use is intended as a private moral stance that ought not be enforced against those not sharing it. The focus, though, is odd, in a context speaking of "use." Publication serves only to disseminate and perhaps to scientifically ratify a study, but primary usage comes as a portion of the scientific enterprise and in contributing to patient care. Once results are known, does it make sense not to use them—and how? By providing inferior treatment? By failing to pursue a suggested hypothesis? By discarding a design for a cold-water suit?

The Arguments

In what follows, I want to concentrate my attention on unpacking one specific argument against using data derived from the Nazi experiments, an argument relying on the symbolic significance of such use. I have reached, in my own mind, a conclusion about this argument: I think it is mistaken, for reasons to be explained. But because this symbolic argument is not ordinarily presented as a distinct reason for rejecting use of the data, I will briefly comment on what appear to be more common arguments for the same conclusion.

Probably the most frequent reason for rejecting use of the Nazi data, one that goes back to General Telford Taylor's arguments before the Nuremberg Tribunal, is that the data represent bad science.[5] The claim is subject to various parsings, other than the threshold denial of the value and validity of the data (discussed above). The claim might be, as Taylor suggested in at least one point, that the results in question could have been demonstrated by bench science, without recourse to human subjects; or, that the results cannot be trusted because the experimenters were untrustworthy; or, that the results cannot be extrapolated to human beings not subjected to Nazi privations and deprivations. All of these arguments, however, are arguments against using poor data (or against the inept use of good data) rather than against Nazi data. The argument would presumably hold as well against poor data collected in an ethically impeccable manner, and so is not an argument specifically relevant to our problem.

The second argument served to ground the decision of editors of medical journals to refuse publication of results achieved through unethical means. The concern here is to deter researchers who would otherwise have a motivation to pursue unethical shortcuts in the interest of their careers. Buttressing this concern is the finding of Barber et al. that "mass producers"—scientists who publish frequently but whose work is rarely cited—as a group hold the most lenient views on the ethics of research.[6] As a deterrence argument, one's reaction will be dominated by one's beliefs about whether the sanction of nonpublication, rather than the sanctions of editorial condemnation, reporting to the granting agency, and so on, is most effective.

My own view is in accord with the nuanced approach of Robert Levine, that individual editorial judgment rather than a uniform approach is most appropriate.[7] At any rate, as a deterrence argument, this seems to me wholly inapplicable to the question of the use of the Nazi data. Evils of the Nazi era, including human experimentation, are many orders of magnitude beyond those that may be deterred by such actions as an eschewal or condemnation of data use.

The Symbolic Arguments

The arguments I would like to focus on are symbolic in nature. They state that science should stand aloof from data derived from a source like the Nazi death camps.

How are we to understand this argument? We are talking of the use of data, not participation in these heinous studies, not replication of atrocities. The wrongs perpetrated were monstrous; those wrongs are over and done. How could the provenance of the data serve to prohibit their use? What ethical structure or theory could, within bounds imposed by logic

and plausibility, ground a relationship between the provenance of the data then, and its use now? I will canvass possibilities, but confess that I remain honestly puzzled by these
questions nonetheless.

It could be felt that by using the data now, the wrong of
which they have grown is retroactively increased. By using
Nazi data, we prolong the Nazi project and perpetuate that
evil. We keep the Nazi project alive, and add an increment,
however small, to its evil.

One response would be that the Holocaust must not be
trivialized by the use of this kind of argument, given the
disparity between the evil of that era and the small modern increment attaching (*ex hypothesi*) to the use of the data.
I respect those who object to this form of trivializing, who
see the *Shoa* ("utter devastation;" the Hebrew term for the
Holocaust) as *sui generis* and therefore prohibit comparisons,
analogies, and extensions; but I do not stand with them. The
Shoa exhausts the ethical ability to imagine evil, but for one
committed to ethics as analysis rather than imagination, this
road cannot be taken. Evil, in my own analytic understanding,
is inexhaustible; the most horrible crime we have experienced
is made worse by adding to it a further wrong, however minor.

My response would therefore come along different lines.
First, the current scientific and medical use of these data is
not an extension of the Nazi project. The use rather causally
depends on that project; the project has perished, the remaining
detritus has been coopted for another purpose, one that is in
fact quite antithetical to the intentions of the Nazis.

Furthermore, if contemporary actions can retroactively
alter the ethical significance of past actions, the alteration,
in principle, must be capable of going in both directions. There
are some who indeed say that the data *must* be used, for such
use has redemptive values. This is the view that, extended
somewhat, underlies talk about "salvaging some good from
the ashes." I am troubled by this view. Is the wrong diminished, diminishable, in any way whatsoever, because of good
that is mined from it afterward? Were the lives of those sac-

rificed, those *korbanot*, in some need of redemption, so that their lives and deaths become infused with significance because of what this has meant to others following them?

I cannot accept the view that later actions causally dependent on the results of the *Shoa* can retroactively alter the ethical significance of that event. At a deeper level, I am concerned here, as elsewhere, about a view of ethics as outside the realm of causality, as a miasma unbound by time that allows the retroactive undoing of past wrongs by a later consent, or a withdrawal of data obtained deceptively.[8]

Another symbolic reason why science must stand aloof and not use the Nazi data is the belief that the evil of that time somehow infuses, insufflates, the data; and so we who use them are tainted, rendered unclean, by this contact. One who uses the data demonstrates thereby ethical or metaphysical obtuseness.[9]

I say these words, but I do not understand them. As a philosopher and ethicist, I understand ethical evaluation as it is attached to human actions, not to objects or mathematical representations of objects. In spite of not understanding, though, I have heard this argument—perhaps from within—and so I must respond.

The specific manner in which evil, the Nazi taint, infuses the data will depend on the specific understanding of wherein that taint consists. The project of understanding the Nazi horror is, in my own view, one incumbent upon each person—certainly upon each Jew, by reason of the command upon each individual to remember Amalek.[10] (Another relevant commandment, arguably, is the one requiring each Jew to write a Scroll of the Law.)

For my own part, as described elsewhere,[11] I understand the essence of evil itself to be, in the words of Rabbi Adin Steinsaltz, the "bursting of bounds, that which breaks out and goes beyond" proper limits.[12] Following Robert Proctor, my individual understanding of the unique nature of the Nazi evil is put with spare understatement as "Germany carried to an extreme policies that were present in milder forms in other countries."[13] This essence of lack of proportion is a form of evil that cannot suffuse data; it is indeed a form of evil expressed in one who unthinkingly recoils in horror from the use of data, whatever the consequences of that rejection might be.

In my own understanding of the Nazi evil, therefore, the Nazi taint does not contaminate the data; and even if it had, it would not follow that the data may not be used. This specific form of evil was common to all aspects of Nazi society, including the operation of science and research, medicine, the political process, the judiciary, and ethics itself.[14]

Robert Lifton writes, for example, of Dr. R, who participated as a psychiatrist in the Nazi murder of mental patients. His conscience is eased—and his later defense in the dock is buttressed—when his chief tells him, before he begins, of "its theological justification by a particular Catholic priest who had stated that 'euthanasia' was morally justifiable in certain cases."[15] Dr. Joachim Mrugowsky, who was later hanged at Nuremberg for his part in distributing Zyklon B, wrote an introduction to a 19th century volume on medical ethics that the Nazis reprinted to justify their cause.[16]

Many people have noted the progression from writings on euthanasia and eugenics to the Nazi programs of forced sterilization, castration, and murder, with their associated research activities. Like a snowball gathering momentum down a slope, the original core of writings by physicians, lawyers, and philosophers may be discerned in the Holocaust itself. The metaphor is instantiated in the use in extermination camps of the same gassing equipment that had been assembled for mercy killings.

Ethics, therefore, could be perverted to instigate and nurture the Nazi enterprise. Everything can be corrupted. Yet further, ethical reasoning itself could remain active and recognizable in the midst of Nazi activity, and not simply appear as a distorted remnant. Dr. Karl Brandt was another hanged at Nuremberg. Lifton reconstructs Brandt's reasoning process from his testimony at the trials concerning the decision to euthanize psychiatric patients by gassing rather than by narcotics:[17]

"Brandt recalled not liking the idea because he felt that 'this whole question can only be looked at from a medical point of view,' and that 'in my medical imagination carbon monoxide had never played a part.' Killing by gas, that is, made it more difficult to maintain a medical aura. Brandt was able to change his mind when he recalled a personal experience of carbon monoxide poisoning in which he lost consciousness 'without feeling anything', and realized that carbon monoxide 'would be the most humane form of death.' Yet he remained troubled because that method required 'a whole change in medical conception', and gave the matter extensive thought 'in order to put my own conscience right.' He brought up to Hitler the difference of opinion about the two methods, and later remembered the Fuhrer asking, 'Which is the more humane way?' 'My answer was clear,' Brandt testified..."

I had put this down in my notes for this chapter as "a parody of an ethical reasoning process," but that is wrong. This is ethical reasoning itself: ethics turned toward monstrous ends.

If courts may be corrupted, shall we do without courts; if ethical reasoning has been corrupted, what should follow? In my eyes, therefore, the lesson of the *Shoa* is: Everything can be corrupted; only in balance is there salvation.

However, I do not mean to enforce my understanding of the Nazi horror upon others; that is indeed my point. I cannot see how anyone could feel so confident of having accomplished the task of capturing the essential Nazi evil as to derive normative implications from that project, if those implications are used to judge or govern the conduct of others. The second view, therefore, that the data are suffused with the Nazi taint, may only apply in the realm of conscience to those scientists whose individual understandings of the Nazi project entail this result. The result cannot be enforced upon those with a different understanding of that which was unique to the Nazi enterprise.

A third version of the symbolic argument holds that the data need to be suppressed to make a statement. Ethics is serious business, and by refusing to use the Nazi data—by invoking this ultimate scientific sanction—we reinforce how seriously we are prepared to take ethical violations. On the contrary, for that matter, by using the data, we would be stating that we are not prepared to enforce our ethical convictions.

This version presupposes what needs to be proven, namely, that the use of the data—as opposed to the manner of its acquisition—is wrong. Moreover, to make a statement you make a statement, you don't fail to make a statement. Silence is ambiguous and often amounts to the uncomfortably averted gaze, whether consciously intended or not. Statements about the Nazi evil need to be made, in detail, repeatedly, and explicitly, rather than by the indirection of omitting use of the data.

(It may be necessary to distinguish the question currently under examination, Are you necessarily saying anything about the event by using the data? from the quite different question, Is there a duty to say anything about the event when using the data? To that question, the answer must be yes. Even a ritualized, stereotyped condemnation of the Nazi experience, invoked when using the data, is preferable to the bland use of data without acknowledgment, or more likely, to the uncomfortably averted gaze.)

A fourth and final parsing of the notion that science must stand aloof from the Nazi era by not using the Nazi data is that by using the data, one would necessarily be saying something about the event, by way of excuse or mitigation, or even simply by admitting the events of that era within human history and the scope of potential behavior.

This argument is similar to several previously examined, but it is different in one crucial respect. In the view I am now examining, by using the data one does not join oneself to the Nazi project, nor does one intentionally take any symbolic stance concerning that era; nonetheless, one is necessarily *seen by others*—even, if you like, *misconstrued* by others—as saying that the events of that time are not so hideous that they must be bracketed off from all future human experience. The argument maintains that by using the data, one

is perforce *legitimating* those experiments; just as, it could
be argued in another context, by transplanting human fetal
tissue one is necessarily legitimating the abortion that made
that tissue available.[18]

Yet could it be that one is necessarily saying one thing
about the *Shoa*, in using the data, contrary to one's own
intention and motivation? A moral universe such as our own
must, I think, rely on the authors of their own actions to be
primarily responsible for attaching symbolic significance to
those actions. In particular, in this case, I think such an
attribution is impossible; for in using the Nazi data, physicians and scientists are acting pursuant to their own moral
commitment to aid patients and to advance science in the
interest of humankind. The use of data is predicated upon
that duty, and it is in seeking to fulfill that duty that the
symbolic significance of the action must be found.

Ethical Analysis and the Use of the Data

I think this last point may, in fact, be ethically conclusive in
justifying the use of the data when medically or scientifically
indicated otherwise. An illustrative anecdote is related concerning one scion of the Soloveichik rabbinic dynasty who
had permitted violating the Sabbath on behalf of a mildly ill
Jew. Upbraided by his students for having issued such a per-
missive ruling of Jewish law, he responded that in his decision he by no means was taking the laws of the Sabbath
lightly. Rather, he was taking the conflicting duties of
pikuach nefesh, preserving life and health, very seriously.

That concludes the ethical analysis, but something must
be said after analysis is done. I share the discomfort that
many hearing or reading these words must feel, at what
seems like a cold, logical, analytic approach to a topic that
requires appropriate emotion. Discussions on the question
of the use of Nazi data are often infused with passion. This
is understandable, natural, and appropriate, and the absence
of passion—as in my above comments—is disquieting. I could

justify this quality of my remarks by pointing to my own
proper professional role; I write as I have been invited: as
an analytic philosopher and ethicist. A deeper justification,
however, can be offered.

The relationship between reason and emotion in ethical
judgment is controverted and murky. I would not care to try
and resolve it here.[19] But a conclusion on the relationship
between the two is not needed—nor would it even be helpful—
in this context. Here, there is no clear opposition between
the two, with reason without reason arguing for the use
that passion eschews; rather, there are conflicting pulls of
sources both in emotion and in logic, on either side of the
debate. Conflict introduces an asymmetry between reason
and passion, for reason of its essence can adjudicate conflict
as emotion of its essence cannot. In such a case of multileveled
conflict, reason is ultimately necessary in guiding our paths
through the thicket of conflicting claims as well as emotions
involved in this discussion.

All of these claims must be heard, and all legitimate perspectives duly spoken and, finally, weighed by reason. I say
this not because I or other academics have a *right* to speak
of the filthy history of human research during the *Shoa*. That
right may be possessed by survivors, and is certainly possessed by survivors of research; that right is possessed by
them alone. But I, in common with other academics—in common with humankind—indeed labor under a *duty* to speak of
these matters. There is no escaping that responsibility.

Further Reflections
on "Salvaging Good from the Ashes"

This metaphor, in its pure form, creates in the mind's
eye an image of a family whose home and possessions have
been destroyed by fire, sifting through the ashes for something that remains intact; something of value; something that
will help get them through the difficult times that are ahead;
something that bridges their past and their future.

The fire has come—how? We don't know, we have not been told. It stands for us, therefore, as just a fire—a catastrophe, a random tragedy. Fire occupies a special place within the memory of our own species, and, perhaps, of others: the external, blind threat, consuming all in its path, touched off by lightning, itself paradigmatic of capricious harm. This force of nature has by chance struck at the most private space of the family, laying waste their previous labor and present hopes. It is *their* tragedy. In sifting through the ashes, their tragedy is reinforced. But perhaps something good will be found, if only, perhaps, acceptance of loss. The image is simple, self-justifying, and poignant. Its moral force is vitiated when it is invoked of a situation that departs from the metaphor's scenario in some way; and some departures distort it in obscene ways. Yet the metaphor is at most a means of argument, a way to see if an action is justified. Even when apt, it is not itself a justification but only serves to point to a justification. When off the mark, by whatever margin, it points away from some justification, but does not thereby demonstrate an absence of alternative justification.

The metaphor is frequently invoked in discussion of family consent to cadaveric transplantation. Death has struck at random, frequently without warning. (The causes of death most likely to leave organs in transplantable conditions include motor vehicle accidents, violence, and suicide; lightning strikes of the contemporary scene.) Chance happening is, for this family, intimate tragedy. Organ donation forces them to confront this tragedy, and it may help them to master it. Alter the circumstances somewhat, and the isomorphism with the metaphor becomes uncertain. We presume the closeness of families, but know this is not always so. A spouse has been recently separated under bitter circumstances: Is he responding to a tragedy *of his* in "donating" his wife's organs?

Anecdotally, it is common for expectant couples who have been informed that their fetus is anencephalic to ask whether the organs may be transplanted, to salvage good from this tragedy. What meaning does this have for them? Is this request a means of coping with tragedy, or a denial or tragedy? Is the request motivated by a previous close bonding with the expected child, or by a wish to create future distance? Yet, does it necessarily matter, in the end? Both motivations are rooted in normal parental feelings, worthy—if not equally worthy—of respect.

The metaphor, as applied to the *Shoa*, is particularly strained. Above all else, the Holocaust was neither a harm nor a catastrophe: It was an evil wreaked by moral agents who should be held responsible for murder. Its ashes speak of arson. The scientists sifting through the data are neither victims nor the agents of victims. They are at best, insofar as this metaphor is concerned, curious onlookers. Those who use the data unreflectively and without attribution may be vandals of the site. Some German scientists who continued their career thereafter are criminals themselves who never left the intellectual scene of their crime. For these reasons, I firmly reject the idea that the Nazi data may or must be used to salvage good from the ashes. To say this, however, is to deny a form of justification, not to deny justification itself. For the very distinct reason argued in my paper, I believe some use of the Nazi data is justified.

From: *When Medicine Went Mad* Ed.: A. Caplan
©1992 The Humana Press Inc.

Can Scientists Use Information Derived from the Concentration Camps?

Ancient Answers to New Questions

Velvl W. Greene

Introduction

The style used for writing an essay—the format for con-
veying thoughts—is never as important as the thoughts themselves. Still, at the very outset, I am confronted with a style
dilemma: Should I try to analyze the Nazi data issue using a
subjective "first person" format—full of "I" and "my"—or
should I, instead, revert to the classic "third person" style
with its editorial "we" and more somber phraseology? The
first lends itself better to emotional descriptions of human
tragedy and passionate debate about its consequences. But
editors of scientific journals and philosophical treatises seem
to prefer the more formal approach, which dampens passion.
Third person styles project images of reasoned objectivity and
academic authority. They can be used to describe suffering
without breaking into tears. They might be able to deal with
the Holocaust without going mad.

The style dilemma may appear to be trivial. It may
dilute and distract from the real dilemma—whether the possible benefit of the Nazi data to medicine, science, and those
whom medicine and science serve today outweighs the potential

danger of justifying the Nazi experiments and desecrating the memory of the Holocaust victims. But in its way, it is a paradigm of that deeper issue: Can we view the Holocaust objectively or are the nerve endings still too raw? Can we—may we—analyze the Holocaust and the Nazi medical experiments in a rational fashion, and philosophically seek real or embryonic parallels in today's bioethics? Should we evaluate the utilitarian pros and cons of using the Nazi data, academically, or shall we subjectively and emotionally agree with the survivors: "Those weren't experiments; that wasn't research; there are no data; let the victims rest in peace; enough!"?

This dilemma—the equally frustrating choice of being objective or being subjective—permeates every debate on this issue and influences my every attempt to come to grips with the issue. I am a Jew who was old enough "then" to have been "there." I am a vicarious survivor. Only the accident of my birth in Canada instead of where my parents originated distinguishes me from the victims and the survivors. Thus, I have some very subjective feelings about the Holocaust. On the other hand, as a former benchtop researcher in the biomedical sciences, I not only identify with the motives of anyone who wants to advance his own studies, but reject, in principle, any arbitrary attempts to censor or ban data published 40 years ago. As a teacher of medicine and a practitioner of public health, I know the compulsion to save life—immediately or remotely, now or in some distant future—at any cost. But as one who accepts the discipline of Torah in my personal life, I also understand that compulsions, even noble ones, must often be curbed and that slippery moral slopes should be avoided rather than tested.

Perhaps the best that I can do, therefore, in place of providing a brilliant analysis of and ultimate solution for the Nazi data issue is to describe my journeys to both horns of the dilemma and to all the points in between. Ultimately, I will try to summarize the issue as I see it, with the full realization that any compromise satisfies absolutely no one and is probably the only agency that unites all antagonists for the first time—against the compromiser.

The Personal Retrospective
of a Biomedical Researcher

When the original controversy about using the Nazi hypothermia data was examined in the public media, remarkably few interviews were elicited from actual laboratory researchers. That is really too bad. Philosophers, theologians, journalists, and policy makers certainly have much that is valuable to contribute to the debate. But very few really understood the mindset and motivations of the laboratory researcher (Dr. Robert Pozos) whose questions started the debate. Whether or not his documented rationalization for citing Rascher's Dachau experiments was valid is not relevant at the moment. I understood exactly how Dr. Pozos felt because I once stood in his shoes and probably will again.

I did not use Nazi data, but I certainly had access (doesn't everyone?) to other "tainted" data that I felt were extremely useful to my own investigations but that had been developed by others in studies considered immoral, or illegal, or just generally shameful. Some of those studies weren't even very good science and maybe they should have been suppressed— by editors, colleagues, or the researchers themselves. No matter, they became available in one form or another and in my eyes, at that time, they were useful. Perhaps they couldn't be cited as references, but as one of my graduate students often remarked, "The data may be lousy, but they are the only data we have!"

I never used any Nazi data in my own work but I spent a portion of my career in biological warfare research. Put aside for now any questions about the inherent morality or immorality of those studies. Sufficient to say that we were engaged in a "cold war" and I didn't work in the "aggressor" branch. I did the more noble studies, the ones related to defense and to human protection.

Among other things we needed were data on infectious doses: How many microbes were required to initiate an infection? There were many animal studies available, but extrapolation from animal models to humans is fraught with uncertainty;

we were not able to validate the usefulness of our protection devices. In our eyes, it was literally a matter of life and death.

We were legally restrained from doing human experiments. I don't know if I would have participated even had we gotten permission. It was a long time ago and I can't recall exactly what my moral status was then. But I do remember reading through the classified captured documents from the Japanese "731" team, which had done biological experiments on prisoners of war. Their data didn't help much. But I did review them. (I don't recall any sleepless nights; the Japanese didn't experiment on Jews and relatives.)

I recall very clearly how I felt about 10 years ago, when I read *Doctors of Infamy* by Mitscherlich and Mielke for the first time. Several chapters in that book describe the horrible infectious disease experiments carried out by the Nazis in Buchenwald, Natzweiler, and those other hells. When I started reading, I remember feeling horror, anger, and dismay. But as I continued reading, I became engulfed by curiosity. That was the frightening thing! After so many years, my curiosity as a scientist overwhelmed all other emotions (about Jews and relatives) and I kept looking for answers that would have helped my ancient research. I have no doubt, now, that if I had known about that book 30 years ago, I would have cited the Nazi data, looked for more, and used them in the work I was doing.

This absolutely necessary and fundamental curiosity of the good researcher and his constant search for clues that will help his current work are not emphasized sufficiently in the media debates surrounding the Nazi data controversy. I wasn't working in Nazi Germany, nor was Dr. Pozos. We weren't being asked to conduct inhuman experiments. In fact, the work I was doing and the work he is doing now can actually be classified as humanitarian—if successful, we can save lives! Are we seriously being asked to turn a blind eye to information that might be helpful? Are we seriously being told to sublimate our curiosity? It is hard to explain to the layman, even to the philosopher, how the motives and methodology of applied research generate a kind of scientific morality in which the greatest good is a "breakthrough."

The average investigator is confronted with deadlines, on the one hand, and huge chunks of missing data, on the other. Nature does not willingly part with her secrets, and the scientist, if he is any good, is always struggling with unknowns. His struggle is sometimes rewarded with tiny slivers, incremental fragments of knowledge, some of which might advance his progress, but most of which are of no immediate use. Is it fair, Dr. Pozos asks (and so do I) to deliberately ignore previous work that might help in this struggle?

Ask the doctoral candidate whose dissertation research on syphilis could be shortened by a year or even six months if she would use data from the Tuskeegee study. Ask the young assistant professor whose career depends on publications whether he would deny himself access to the excellent pellagra data obtained from inmates of Southern prisons and poor farms, the excellent immunization data obtained by aerosolizing live viruses in Russian classrooms, or the excellent hepatitis data obtained by deliberately infecting retarded children in New York.

Obviously, none of the preceding examples of human experimentation are remotely related to what took place at Dachau, Auschwitz, and Nordhausen. The motives of the experimenters, their methodology, and their concern for the test subjects were in different worlds. I am not even implying equivalence. But I am trying to make the point that to ask an investigator to overlook and ignore data that he deems potentially useful to his work is the equivalent of asking the thirsty desert wanderer to deny himself a drink of water in an oasis where the well was dug by slave labor. Moral considerations might prevail, but don't bet on them.

Dealing with Nazi Data

Possible Scenarios

I don't think any moral argument would have dissuaded me then. After all, I was doing important research and this was a chance to save time and effort. What would happen now, after the public debates and my exposure to the views of the philosophers and theologians? I don't honestly know. Maybe my resolve to pursue the "literature search" would be weakened by the impassioned pleas of the survivors. Maybe I could be convinced by moral reasoning.

If faced with the same dilemma today, I might try, before making a decision, to do some thinking about trade-offs, about gain and loss, about weighing the costs of using the data against the costs of ignoring them.

Essentially, three possible scenarios come to mind:

An Absolute Ban on the use of the data: Either destroying them completely, employing criminal sanctions against their use, or giving them a security classification that essentially removes them from reasonable accessibility.

A Laissez Faire or Libertarian Approach: Ignoring the source and treating the information like any other archival knowledge; whoever takes the time and has the ingenuity to dig it up can use it. The only restrictions would be those imposed by investigators and publishers on their own; very much like what is being done now.

A Selected Suppression or Utilitarian Approach: Developing guidelines and appointing screening committees that will decide who gets access to what and on what basis; to be modeled on our current hospital ethics committees who can deliberate matters of urgency, priority, justice, beneficence, academic freedom, and so forth.

Each of these three approaches will have a different impact on different "populations at risk:"

- The victims of the Nazi experiments and their survivors;
- The perpetrators of the Nazi experiments and their survivors;
- Society today, including researchers, medical professionals, and those who might benefit from the findings;
- Future societies, including potential perpetrators and potential victims.

It is actually possible to prepare a matrix contingency table and to speculate on how each proposed data-handling scenario would influence each population at risk. For example, a complete ban on Nazi data will preserve the autonomy and dignity of the victims and deny any "research credit" to the Nazis. But it might dim the memory of what the Nazis actually did. It might interfere somewhat with current advances in certain types of research, but probably will not be a critical handicap. It might be a deterrent to future Nazi-type unethical experiments, but only if the potential future perpetrators recognize the parallel between themselves and the Nazis and if their primary motivation is to be cited in the literature. It might save some future victims, but again, only if the potential perpetrators are sensitive to world opinion and historical excoriation. It is quite evident that a complete ban on the data will have its greatest impact on researchers and historians; it will satisfy the pleas of the victims and survivors, but it will not do much else for a world that really does not know and cares even less about what happened in Mengele's barracks 45 years ago.

The same kind of analysis for each of the other scenarios would yield a similar variety of simultaneous outcomes that can also be ranked on some type of gain-loss scale for each of the populations at risk. Thus, the laissez faire approach might provide some benefit to society and to current medicine, but those benefits must be balanced against the message that there are no objective moral standards in science. The establishing of such moral standards by the Selected Suppression model would be paid for by bureaucratic delays and inhibition of research incentive. No single approach has a clear advantage over the other.

Slippery Slopes Exist on Many Mountains

Even though the words have become cliches in contemporary ethics debates, we are actually dealing with several classical slippery slopes, e.g., the danger that legitimizing the use of Nazi data would ultimately legitimize the experiments themselves, e.g., if we do not absolutely reject the data obtained from those whom the Nazis defined as "subhuman" we must sooner or later lend credence to those who destroy or perform experiments on fetuses whom they define as subhuman. The concerns about sliding down these slopes are legitimate and should not be arbitrarily dismissed. However, it should be pointed out as a matter of fact that there are plenty of other icy mountains down which societies, professions, and individuals can slide even if their intention is really to climb higher or even just to stand still while catching a breath.

Banning access to data because of pleas from the victims or because a tribunal decides that the data were derived from cruel and immoral experiments smells faintly like the smoke of burning books that were written by cruel and immoral authors. It is not really a bad smell at first. There are excellent reasons for burning some of the trash that is published, just as there are excellent reasons for sealing the Nazi records. If we could just stop at banning the Nazi data we might be willing to pay the current cost of handicapping some current research projects. But, to paraphrase Heine's immortal warning about burning books and burning people, a society that burns Nazi data will soon go on to burn other data that will be deemed in the future as equally excoriable. What will be next after Rascher's notes and Mengele's reports? South African medical journals look like good candidates. What is to stop student vigilantes who dictate investment and disinvestment policies to intimidated Boards of Regents from banning library acquisitions from Soweto and Azerbaijan and Valparaiso and Tel Aviv? Each of these bans would find eager supporters among those constituencies who want to "purify" our minds and "punish" evil. Should we, in the name of ethics, create a precedent, a push down a slippery slope?

The Selected Suppression approach sounds good and can be implemented. Systems for classifying research data are already in place to protect the national security. All we would have to do is include the Nazi data at a certain high level and assign quantitative access numbers to different investigators, based on how many lives the research is designed to save, which agency is sponsoring the research, the short- or long-term payoffs, and so on. This kind of system will become the darling daughter of institutional and governmental bureaucracy, and will function parallel to Affirmative Action offices, compulsory bussing programs, continuing education credits, and institutional review boards. It will probably degenerate into the same swamp that the other programs share: lots of clerks, lots of printouts to show that we are in conformance with some kind of guidelines, and a general feeling that it must be doing some good or why is it still hanging around.

There is even a side slope with its own little precipice that trails off from the Selected Suppression slide. It is the reality that any kind of data suppression will ultimately punish the "good soldier" who obeys the law and will reward the smart, the sneaky, and the scofflaw who knows how to manipulate the system. Bootleggers make their greatest piles during prohibition.

The most frightening slope—perhaps because its terminus and pitch is unknown—is that of the Laissez Faire or Libertarian or Status Quo approach. We simply do not trust ourselves or our colleagues to do the proper thing when it comes to self-regulation and self-restraint. We see how human the doctor and the field scientist really are, we know the mix of motives and ambitions that fuel their efforts, and we are afraid that they will not make the "right" decision about which data to use and how they should be used and how they should be cited. We know that nonethical research is a current fact and feel that Nazi-type research is still a possibility.

Nonetheless, the unknown slope associated with free access and exchange of information might still be preferable to the ones we know will lead to disaster: the dangers of a complete ban or the convolutions of a selected ban. Obviously, our difficulty is with the doctors and the researchers and not with the data. If we need a better system of selecting medical students or granting doctorates, then we should tend to it. If there is a deficiency in the moral education of our researchers, let us rectify it. Because we did not, in the past, prevent the Holocaust and the Nazi "research," we want to compensate by banning or controlling the data that emanated. Self-delusion might be the most slippery and most dangerous slope of all.

Principles of Jewish Medical Ethics Relevant to the Issue

This section should have been written first, if only because it might provide the clearest guidelines to the Nazi data dilemma. But unyielding deontological solutions are not too readily accepted in either the emotional, subjective world nor its utilitarian, objective counterpart. Consequently, it was thought advisable to sketch first some of the snares and slippery slopes that exist on the other paths that might be followed.

As a Jew, I believe that God not only created the universe, He provided guidance and a rather well worked out body of instructions to humankind. In this view, there are no unanswerable questions about "what" to do under certain circumstances. There might be a lot of speculation as to "why," but action guidelines to the query "Can we use the Nazi data?" will be found by consultation with rabbinical authorities who are intimately familiar with the Talmud and the Codes of Jewish Law and the thousands of years of Rabbinic responsa, i.e., Jewish Medical Ethics.[1]

This is not the place for a thumbnail sketch of the responsa system or for any apologies regarding its use. Suffice to say that when confronted with an issue as profound and passionate as that posed by this problem, I did whatever research I could to establish the facts and then queried several rabbis learned in this particular field.

A specific and satisfactory answer to my query, however, was difficult to find. There is a growing body of responsa on questions of the Holocaust and there is a world of Halakhic literature on medicine. But the specific subject of Nazi data and whether we can use it in medicine and biomedical research today, has not been analyzed by any rabbinic authority. Our rabbis refrain from theoretical speculations in their

Halakhic writings; it appears that a specific case has not yet been presented for judicial decision before any of the scholars capable of dealing with such matters. As a consequence, the rabbis I consulted were just able to present several well established principles and precedents that might have some bearing on the issue. This is similar to asking a good attorney for his opinion about secular law on an issue that has not yet been tested in court. His opinion will be based on previous rulings made in parallel or related cases, on constitutional statutes, on legislative acts; but it is not really "law" until tried in court and validated during the appeals process.

The most important principle of Jewish Medical Ethics that pertains to the possible use of Nazi data is the principle of *Pikuach Nefesh* or saving a human life. This is a primary responsibility for every man but is particularly incumbent on physicians who have unique skills and knowledge. In the view of Halakha, the physician acting as a healer is considered to be a special agent and partner of the Almighty. His professional judgment about the suitability of medical treatment is more important than his piety. When involved in life-saving acts, his medical judgments carry more weight than most of the 613 commandments in the Torah.

The preservation of life is a fundamental religious commandment that takes precedence over every other divine precept except under three defined circumstances: when the life-saving activity involves murder, idolatry, or sexual immorality. A physician engaged in *Pikuach Nefesh* is obligated to desecrate the Sabbath, to transgress the immutable dietary laws, to force-feed a patient on Yom Kippur, to break the laws of confidentiality, even to lie to the patient—as long as in his professional opinion the action will contribute toward the saving of human life. Moreover, if the physician possesses some life-saving remedy or knowledge, refusal to use it would be tantamount to bloodshed.

The Halakha, in innumerable instances, distinguishes between acts that are forbidden *a priori* and the consequences of acts that are already *ex post facto*. If a forbidden act cannot be undone or reversed, the restrictions on deriving some benefit from the act, particularly if the benefits involve healing, are much less stringent. Thus, for example, it is forbidden to steal a medicine. But if a physician thinks he can heal a patient with a medicine that he knows has been stolen and that cannot be returned, he is usually given permission to use that medicine.

The rules about knowledge—in distinction to things—that may be acquired under questionable circumstances are even more liberal. The Halakha makes it very clear that if there is a choice between two physicians, one an observant Jew with no special competence, and the other completely unobservant, or even a heathen idolator, who might not have observed all the moral scruples while studying, but who is now an expert in diagnosis and therapy, you must choose the second!

One more principle of Jewish Medical Ethics that bears relevance to the discussion: Judaism teaches that man is created in the image of God. Thus, the physical body, the vessel of the soul, is considered inviolate and must be extended every dignity even after the soul departs. Jewish Law does not sanction routine autopsies. They are permitted only in those cases where an immediate and urgent need exists for information essential to the treatment of other patients. Even then, to avoid desecration of the body or "benefiting from the dead," the postmortem examination is performed under very restricted and scrupulous conditions. But, there is no absolute ban on autopsies. If, in the physician' s opinion, the life of another human being can be saved or a deadly disease can be prevented, then permission for an autopsy should be granted. Similar Halakhic rulings have recently been issued with respect to authorizing donations of organs for transplantation.

It is quite evident, from the principles cited above, that rabbinic permission to use 45-year old data would probably be granted to any physician who can make a case that the information is pertinent to saving the life of his patient. The data were gathered illegally, by inhuman murderers, and in indescribably horrible circumstances. The world that witnessed (and tolerated!) those experiments should have been dissolved in the waters of Noah or incinerated by the fire and sulfur of Sodom. But it wasn't, and we are obligated to continue living and obeying the will of God. If the use of Nazi data today does not involve committing murder, worshipping idols, or illicit sex, its use for *Pikuach Nefesh* cannot be denied.

It should be emphasized, however, that this anticipated rabbinic ruling might not be directly applicable to the hypothermia research of Dr. Pozos. There are parallels, to be sure, but there are also sufficient differences between *Pikuach Nefesh* and biomedical research to generate a reasonable atmosphere of doubt. The arguments cited above deal with direct benefit, with the here and now, with life and death, and with physicians' opinions. Under these circumstances, the rulings go beyond "permission" and sometimes become "obligation." But the Halakha might say that since advancing biomedical knowledge provides only doubtful and delayed benefits for future patients who are as yet unknown, research is not, itself, a sufficient reason to risk desecration of a martyr's memory or justification of a murderer. More important, since the data are old and of very questionable quality, considering the "scientific" standards that prevailed in the camps, an even greater shadow of doubt is cast on their potential benefit. Under these circumstances, the case for using the Nazi data becomes more and more ambiguous. Whether or not the potential benefit to life-saving practices of the future is of sufficient import, and whether denying a researcher access to data is equivalent to preventing a physician from exercising his professional judgment— these cannot be answered by speculation and must await an authoritative responsum from a recognized scholar.

Perhaps the conflict between the "need" of the researcher and the "plea" of the Holocaust survivor can be found in the following Hasidic aphorism: "What one is obligated to do, he must do with enthusiasm; what one is forbidden to do, be must avoid completely; what one is just 'permitted' to do, it may be better if he just doesn't do it."

From the Specific to the General

The use of Nazi data issue will probably resolve itself with no external bans or selective bans. The history of biomedical research and the attitudes of those engaged in it suggests that those who still need the information will find a way to use it. If public opinion and editors insist on precautions to preserve the dignity of the martyrs or to prevent justifying the perpetrators, then an appropriate system of citation and editorial footnotes will be developed. Time itself, as well as the quality of the data, will act to diminish their importance to current research. After all, how many citations in the biomedical literature are older than 10 years? Ironically, in the future, the only ones who will be citing the data will be those who intend to show why it should not be used—historians, ethicists, and theologians. The bigger issue is the double danger that the Nazi experiments and experimenters will become either oversensationalized or that they will become trivialized. In the first instance, the cruelty and bestiality and horror will place the Holocaust and the Nazi experiments beyond comprehension. They will stand so unique—a onetime historical aberration—so inhuman that no human can grasp it. It will become of legendary importance as a legend, but with little relevance to real life.

Horrible as it was, the Holocaust might not have been the worst example of the bestiality to which man may sink. Who judges these cruelty olympics, anyway, and what criteria do you use to rank Attila the Hun vs Ivan Demjanjuk vs Tomas Torquemada? The Holocaust is not even the best historical example of the dangers of "redefinition." The Germans redefined Jews and Slavs and Gypsies as subhuman so Rascher could use them as "test subjects." But redefinition of people and individuals as different, inferior, enemies, uncivilized, or heathen is historically and currently common. Once redefined, these new species are fair targets for killing, conquest, exploitation, colonialization, or conversion to the true faith—or all of these at once.

At the other end of the spectrum is the possibility that
Nazi experiments will simply be equated to unethical medical
practices. Look what has happened to those other Holocaust
memories: "Ghetto" today is almost a universal synonym for
slum, with no shred of reference to either the misery or the
heroism the word evokes; "genocide" is used by any politician in or out of the United Nations to refer to any military
action his side is losing.

The Nazi data issue must not be allowed to become sen-
sationalized beyond credibility or dissipated as a historical
model. The issue is not one of semantics or medical ethics or
scientific reliability. It is not a question of tainted, immoral,
and illegal data. It is rather tainted, immoral, and illegal
humans who did the work—people very much like us.

The Holocaust stands unique in the long annals of human
degradation because so many civilized, educated, "god-
fearing," and culturally advanced human beings perpetrated
it, enjoyed it, benefited from it, and watched it happen. The whole
civilized world was involved, both inside and outside the
camps, both inside and outside Germany, and all over the
world. And neither they nor we did very much to stop it from
happening while there was still time.

The Holocaust addresses particularly the cultured and
the educated, everyone who is presently involved in biomedical research and practice, in engineering and administration and technology. Are we different from Rascher,
Gebhardt, Hirt, and Grawitz? Do we deserve the honor and
dignity that we claim as a prerequisite of our profession?

I submit that we must put the Holocaust and the Nazi
experiments directly under the floodlights and on center stage
even if some of us and our past and present are partly illu-
minated by the glare. Instead of banning the Nazi data or
assigning it to some archivist or custodial committee, I
maintain that it be exhumed, printed, and disseminated to
every medical school in the world along with the details of
methodology and the names of the doctors who did it, whether
or not they were indicted, acquitted, or hanged. It should be

taught in the medical school classrooms, not during a special course in ethics or history, but as part of the anatomy, physiology, pathology, microbiology, and pharmacology portion of the curriculum. The data should be presented regularly during grand rounds and research symposia. Let the students and the residents and the young doctors know that this was not ancient history or an episode from a horror movie where the actors get up after filming and prepare for another role. It was real. It happened yesterday. It was "medical;" it was "scientific;" it was contemporary with the development of penicillin!

They tried to burn the bodies and to suppress the data. We must not finish the job for them. Personally, I will never look at another Petri dish in my laboratory without remembering how they made bacteriological culture media in Auschwitz from human flesh. I submit that this is an appropriate use of the Nazi data.

We might never fully understand "why" and "how," but at least we can remember "what." That is what the victims and their survivors asked. We should also remember our colleagues who did it and our close cultural and professional affinity to them. That is what the world of medicine needs. It is really a "first person" type of thing.

From: *When Medicine Went Mad* Ed.: A. Caplan
©1992 The Humana Press Inc.

Medical Killing and Euthanasia

Then and Now

Which Way Down the Slippery Slope?

Nazi Medical Killing and Euthanasia Today

Ruth Macklin

A Troubling Case

A case that came before a recent meeting of a hospital ethics committee was troubling, but not uncommon. The patient, about 70 years old, had been brought to the emergency room with a fever of 107°. Following her admission to the hospital seven months earlier, she was given a diagnosis of "status epilepticus." Now she is in the Intensive Care Unit, on a respirator from which she cannot be weaned. Brain damage is far-reaching. The doctors are having difficulty gaining access for the insertion of intravenous lines. The patient does not respond to stimuli, has already developed large decubitus ulcers, and requires regular suctioning and turning. A private duty nurse carries out these tasks of daily maintenance.

The patient's family—her husband and two daughters—were told of the bleak prognosis from the beginning. Yet they insist that this level of care be continued. The husband refuses to consider the physician's suggestion to write a "Do Not Resuscitate Order" for the patient. Contrary to expert medical evaluations, the family believes the patient is communicating with them. They refuse to believe the prognosis and hold out hope that the patient will recover.

I said this case is not uncommon. The relatives of patients often demand treatment beyond the point where physicians are able to prevent death or restore functioning.

Families sometimes maintain false hope—in their grief or denial—that a miracle will occur. Doctors are reluctant to ignore or override the wishes of a patient's family in such cases, not only out of fear of being sued but also out of respect for the next of kin as surrogate decision-makers for patients who lack decisional capacity. One good reason for deferring to family members is that they are the ones most likely to know what the patient would have wanted regarding continuation or cessation of life supports. A less compelling reason, ethically speaking, is that doctors are unwilling to offend family members. When the patient can no longer participate in decisions, it is the family the physician must deal with.

Yet there was a troubling aspect to this case, which was the reason the physician sought the help of the ethics committee. The doctor has been pressured by the hospital administration to discontinue this level of therapy because of financial costs. The hospital is paying for the private duty nurse, and a bed in the ICU costs considerably more than one on a regular hospital floor. The patient is being given antibiotics, as well as artificial food and fluids to maintain her life. The physician believes he should be an advocate for the family of his patient, and that the right course of action is to honor their wishes about the level of care being provided. Yet he is being criticized, even threatened by his superiors for refusing to make financial considerations the overriding factor. The message is clear that this patient is absorbing a disproportionate share of the hospital's resources.

The physician told the ethics committee that the patient and her husband are Holocaust survivors, having spent years in a concentration camp. The family's experience under the Nazis underscores their unwillingness to forgo life-prolonging treatments. Some members of the ethics committee wonder whether it is ethically relevant that these people are Holocaust survivors. No one makes the explicit suggestion that lowering the level of care would constitute euthanasia.

Everyone agrees that continued biological life could not benefit the patient herself. Yet some committee members are deeply worried about the justification for withdrawing treatment. The patient is costing the hospital too much money. She has become a "useless eater."

Would it be an act of euthanasia to deny this patient her private duty nurse and to reduce the level of care by removing her from the ICU? The answer depends on the definition of "euthanasia." Physicians at the ethics committee meeting were in unanimous agreement that the patient's death would be hastened if she received anything less than her current level of care. Yet the intention of lowering the level of care is to save money, not to cause the death of the patient. But her imminent death could be foreseen, even if not directly intended. Nonetheless, death would not relieve the suffering of this patient, since she is unresponsive and the extent of brain damage precludes the possibility of any awareness. However, according to one viewpoint, people who are comatose "are benefited by euthanasia, even though they are not relieved of suffering."[1]

One member of the ethics committee suggested that the family be told that the hospital simply does not have the resources to continue to provide this level of care for this patient. Is the patient's family mistaken in thinking that withdrawal of care bears any resemblance to what happened in Nazi Germany?

Euthanasia Under the Nazis and Today

Three Approaches

No ethical indictment is more devastating than the charge of "Nazi practices." Yet the temptation to issue that indictment often surfaces when euthanasia is mentioned. Although it is hard to remain dispassionate in any discussion relating to the Holocaust, several questions deserve sober reflection: Were there any aspects of the euthanasia program under the Nazis that could legitimately be described as 'euthanasia' in our sense of the term? Is there a clear and unequivocal meaning of the concept of euthanasia today? Are there any relevant similarities between "medical killing" during the Holocaust and recent biomedical practices involving termination of treatment? If there are such similarities, does ethical consistency require that we accept or condemn both?

Three general approaches to this set of questions can be discerned. To be sure, there are differences in style and method among adherents of any one approach. But to understand and analyze the overall debate, it is useful to draw the boundary lines with broad brushstrokes. The first approach finds all too many similarities between the Nazi "euthanasia program" and what goes on in hospitals today. The second approach argues against the meaningfulness and accuracy of alleged similarities. The third approach is not an intermediate position between the first two, but rather, one that sounds a cautionary alarm about the dangers of the slippery slope.

In the first group are those who find current practices involving termination of life-sustaining treatment unacceptable. Some in this group hold that euthanasia, *by definition,* is morally wrong, and that today's practices are all examples of euthanasia. A more nuanced view claims that a great many contemporary biomedical practices have ideological roots similar to those of the Nazis. Proponents of both viewpoints use Nazi allusions and comparisons to buttress their account.

An example of the definitional indictment is an inflammatory article entitled "Hitler's Euthanasia Program—More Like Today's Than You Might Imagine." It begins by asserting: "Today we are faced with the prospect that our society will accept and legalize, the crime of euthanasia, for which Nazi doctors hanged at Nuremberg."[2]

The article uses the phrase "today's Death Lobby" to refer to advocates of patients' right to refuse life-prolonging treatment, and identifies a "whole breed of 'medical ethicists' in the service of death...whose vocation is to tell doctors, hospitals, families and clergymen that it is highly moral to kill helpless patients in American hospitals."[3]

Less inflammatory but nonetheless issuing a similar indictment is an article by Nat Hentoff, who argues that even with the very best of intentions, it is possible "to think and plan in a way that would bring about results that were also the goals of the Nazis—from different motivations."[4] Hentoff picks out several targets. One is Daniel Callahan, for implying in his book, *Setting Limits,* that "the lives of the elderly are worth less—in terms of prolonging them—than other lives," a view Hentoff assimilates to the Nazis' *"lebensunwertes Leben,"* 'life unworthy of life.' "[5] Another target is Ronald Cranford, along with others who argue that when individuals are in a persistent vegetative state, "personhood" has vanished, and "without personhood, there could be no act of murder," that is, wrongful killing.

A lengthy, more nuanced article by Richard John Neuhaus serves as an example of the view that active euthanasia is morally prohibited, and moreover, it is always wrong to withhold or withdraw certain medical treatments. Entitled "The Return of Eugenics," this article argues that Nazi Germany's doctrines and practices "effected but a momentary pause in the theory and practice of eugenics...[T]oday, ...eugenics is back..."[6] Neuhaus asserts that "the question of euthanasia is...an integral part of the progress of the eugenics project."[7] The meaning of 'eugenics' is broadened here to include new ways of using and terminating undesired human life,"[8] as well as other biomedical practices the author deplores. One such practice, abortion, is likened by Neuhaus to the killing of Jews, gypsies, homosexuals, and Slavs by the Nazis.[9] Here, Neuhaus claims that the justifications offered for abortion and research with human embryos in our society "are very much like the arguments employed in the Holocaust..."[10]

The second approach is at the opposite end of the spectrum. Writers in this group seek to deny either definitional equivalence or factual similarities between the Nazis' euthanasia program and today's examples of forgoing life-sustaining treatment.

First is the attempt to sever the very meaning of the concept of euthanasia from the Nazi program that went by that name. In an article whose purpose is simply to define the term 'euthanasia,' Beauchamp and Davidson dismiss an entire range of examples, claiming that "some actions which have commonly been denominated euthanasia—such as the overused Nazi examples—would not be euthanasia on our definition."[11] Seeking to provide a "definition...which dictates no moral conclusions, these authors argue that the concept of euthanasia "includes no inherently evaluative component. 'Murder' entails wrongful killing, and therefore possesses both prescriptive and descriptive force; but 'euthanasia' is not analogous."[12]

Not only is the concept of euthanasia devoid of a negative evaluative component according to this account; it also lacks a positive evaluative component, despite its derivation from the Greek word for "good death." Thus, Beauchamp and Davidson argue, it is not a contradiction to say "an act of euthanasia is immoral."[13] Correctly describing an act as an instance of euthanasia is one thing; evaluating a particular act described as euthanasia is quite another.

Beauchamp and Davidson are correct in observing that the term "euthanasia" need not entail either a positive or a negative evaluation of the act. The concept can be defined and used in a purely descriptive way, denoting a means of bringing about death but neither praising nor condemning it. However, most people who talk or write about euthanasia do not use the term in that purely descriptive way. Beauchamp and Davidson are telling us how people ought to use the concept, what the term euthanasia "really" means. Most people haven't read their scholarly article, though, and will continue to use the term with its built-in value connotations.

A variant of this second approach to the question of comparisons between the Nazi euthanasia program and today's medical practices takes the position that not only do certain concepts used by the Nazis differ in meaning from their current usage; but also, there are great factual dissimilarities between what the Nazis were about and what goes on today.

This denial takes several forms. One focuses not directly on euthanasia, but on other concepts, most notably, "quality of life." In an article entitled " 'Quality of Life' and the Analogy with the Nazis," Cynthia Cohen provides a detailed explication of how the Nazis used that phrase, arguing that their use was radically different from our own. The Nazis viewed the quality of life of individuals only in terms of their social worth, how they were of service to the *Volk*. In contrast, Cohen maintains, "a coherent 'quality of life' position is grounded in a theory of the value of humans as beings with a capacity for self-reflective deliberation and action. It explicates the meaning of 'quality of life' of human beings in terms of standards of individual well-being, rather than in terms of social worth."[14]

Yet even when its meaning is confined to standards of individual well-being, the phrase "quality of life" poses the problem of determining how high or low a standard of individual well-being is acceptable. In a long-standing debate surrounding the ethics of allowing handicapped newborns to die, standards have been proposed that many people consider unacceptably high. An example is the criterion used by John Lorber, a British pediatrician: "The ability to work or marry."[15]

A more direct form of this approach focuses on the term "euthanasia" itself. Such terms, when applied to the Nazi experience "do not have our meaning. These terms and the programs they stood for were integral aspects of Nazi racism. Nazi racism derived from a theory about the ultimate value of the purity of the *Volk*..."[16] This observation, by Lucy Dawidowicz, makes only half of the comparison, however. It fails to specify *our* meaning—assuming that there is a single meaning, which there is not—of the term 'euthanasia.'

The Concept of Euthanasia

Before proceeding to the third approach—one that finds both similarities and differences between the Nazi program and today's practices—this is a suitable place to pause for the obligatory conceptual inquiry. Although there is not a single definition of euthanasia, there is a core meaning com-

mon to a number of leading candidates. To cite only a few of
the definitions that have been offered:

1. "The painless inducement of a quick death;"
2. "An act or practice of painlessly putting to death persons
   suffering from incurable conditions or diseases;"
3. "The intentional putting to death by artificial means of
   persons with incurable or painful disease;"
4. "An act...in which one...kills another person...for the benefit
   of the second person, who actually does benefit from being
   killed."[17]

Not only do these definitions differ substantially from
one another; they also are open to "fatal counterexamples."[18]
Definition 1. could be applied to a simple case of murder, such
as injecting a quick-acting poison into a sleeping person whom
one hates. This definition also permits accidental death to
be an instance of euthanasia.[19] Definition 2. could also be a
simple case of murder, such as injecting a quick-acting poison into a rich relative who has a mild case of multiple scle-
rosis (an incurable disease) without the relative's consent and
for the purpose of inheriting his wealth. Definition 3. includes
the vague and problematic term 'artificial,' and like 1. and
2., also omits mention of the central intention, namely to end
suffering or to benefit the person whose death is intended.
Definition 4. comes closer to our intuitive understanding of
the concept of euthanasia. But cast in terms of one person
killing a second person, it rules out, by definition, situations
in which suffering patients are passively "let die," rather than
actively killed.

One attempt to summarize the relevant differences
between the Nazis' use of the term "euthanasia" and what is
assumed to be our current meaning appears in a historical
study of Nazism.[20] It is worth quoting the long opening paragraph of the chapter entitled "The 'Euthanasia' Programme
1939–1945:"

"In current parlance the term *euthanasia* refers to the
practice of so-called 'mercy killing,' that is of painlessly
ending the life of a person who is terminally ill at his

or her request or, if they are no longer capable of making such a request, then with the consent of their relatives. It is a highly controversial issue, but it should not be confused with the Nazi 'euthanasia' policy. For, although the Nazis used the term to describe their own programme of killing over one hundred thousand mentally sick and handicapped persons from 1939 to 1945, their practice had little in common with the term as it is normally understood. In the first place, the decision to terminate the life of a patient under the Nazi programme was taken not by the individual concerned or by his or her relatives but by an official body. Secondly, the criterion for the 'mercy killing' was not the welfare of the individual patient but whether or not the patient's life was judged to be of 'value' or 'worth,' and of value not to the individual concerned (although the Nazis sometimes used this as an additional justification) but to the community.[21]

The first condition—that the decision to terminate the life of a patient be made either by the individual concerned or by his or her relatives—is not part of the *meaning* of the term 'euthanasia;' nor does it fully and accurately describe current or proposed practices. The second condition—that the criterion for mercy killing be the welfare of the individual patient—does capture the central feature of the concept of euthanasia, but whether or not the sufferer must be terminally ill remains a matter of conceptual and ethical dispute. There is great uncertainty and consequently, much ethical controversy about how to determine the welfare or "best interest" of individuals who are incapable of speaking for themselves.

A classification scheme often used to elucidate the concept of euthanasia distinguishes four categories: Active, passive, voluntary, and involuntary. Each category can be marked by a paradigm case, yet conceptually and practically, these distinctions are easily blurred. In the following examples, assume that the intention in causing the death of the individual is to end suffering or to benefit the patient.

A clear case of active euthanasia is the injection of a lethal substance into a patient with advanced, metastatic cancer, who is suffering extreme pain and discomfort. The act would count as *voluntary*, active euthanasia if the patient knew she was in the advanced stage of incurable cancer, requested the injection, and believed the injection would cause her death. It would be *involuntary*, active euthanasia if the patient were not consulted and her wishes were not known.

Paradigm cases of *passive* euthanasia are ones in which a life-sustaining treatment is withheld. These are cases of "letting die," rather than "killing." A patient who requests to be allowed to die rather than being intubated and placed on a ventilator might be said to seek voluntary, passive euthanasia. The case becomes more convincing as relief of suffering if the patient had already been on a ventilator, found that mode of existence intolerable, and after being weaned requests that she not be reintubated even if necessary to prolong her life. To ensure that death by this means would be painless as well as quick, the patient requests that she be adequately sedated.

An example of involuntary, passive euthanasia would be withholding renal dialysis from an irreversibly comatose patient whose kidneys have failed. The act is involuntary because the patient has not requested that dialysis be withheld. Since on virtually all accounts continued life would not be a benefit to an irreversibly comatose individual, this case could qualify conceptually as euthanasia.

But here is where definitional uncertainty begins, leading to the conceptual debate. Does a "good death" require that the patient be relieved of suffering? Can death itself count as a benefit to a person who is comatose or in a persistent vegetative state? Reasonable people disagree on the answers to these concepual questions, yet without agreement on that point, the boundaries of euthanasia remain fuzzy.

According to one view, patients in a coma or persistent vegetative state (PVS) "are benefited by euthanasia, even though they are not relieved of suffering."[22] An opposing view holds that "no definition [of euthanasia] is acceptable which includes under its instances persons who are comatose..."[23] This is because the concept of euthanasia should apply only in cases where the intent is to benefit a person by relieving that person's suffering. It is important to see this as a conceptual dispute, not an ethical disagreement. There is virtually no controversy over whether individuals who are in a coma or in the unresponsive condition known as PVS are experiencing suffering. Opponents in the conceptual dispute might disagree about whether withholding life supports from comatose individuals counts as euthanasia; yet they may still agree on whether it is morally permissible to forgo the respirator.

Conceptual debate is even more intense when it comes to drawing a line between "active" and "passive" means. Is the removal of life supports already in place active or passive? Many physicians insist that withdrawing treatment counts as "active" euthanasia. They argue that if they fail to institute life-prolonging treatment, it is the disease that kills the patient; but if life supports already in place are withdrawn, it is the doctor who kills the patient. This conceptual maneuver rests on an underlying ethical stance: Allowing to die is morally permissible, but killing is not.

Yet that proposition is problematic. It brings to mind the rationalization used by Nazi doctors involved in the Child Euthanasia Program. Some left their institutions without heat, allowing the children to die of exposure. This enabled the doctors to offer the rationale that they were not engaged in murder, since "withholding care" was simply "letting nature take its course."[24] This shows that ethical permissibility cannot rest simply on whether the means leading to death are "active" or "passive."

Indeed, it is suggested by proponents of active euthanasia that active killing is sometimes more humane, and therefore, more ethically acceptable than allowing to die. When performed under limited, specified circumstances and with adequate safeguards, a painless lethal injection is more humane, they argue, than letting the cancer patient die a slow, agonizing death. Among those who believe that active killing, under certain circumstances, can be ethically permissible are physicians who practice active euthanasia in the Netherlands, along with their supporters; and members of the Hemlock Society in the United States, along with those who signed a petition seeking to place a referendum legalizing active euthanasia on the California ballot in 1988. Both the existing practice in Holland and the proposed plan in California permit only *voluntary* euthanasia, and both require that the patient who requests euthanasia be terminally ill at the time the request is made. Additional safeguards, designed to prevent abuses, are also built into the practice.

At the other extreme are those who oppose any and all withholding of life-sustaining treatment, whether active or passive, voluntary or involuntary; and a more moderate group who draw the moral line at withholding food and fluids, or more generally, at the boundary between "ordinary" and "extraordinary" treatments or "routine" and "heroic" measures. Withholding food and fluids amounts to "starving people to death," it is argued. What could be more like the Nazi euthanasia program?

The Nazi Euthanasia Program

The case that is said to have precipitated the first phase of the Nazi euthanasia program, known as the "children's 'euthanasia' program," occurred in late 1938 or early 1939 and involved a handicapped child. As recalled by Hitler's personal physician, Karl Brandt, in his testimony at the Nuremberg Medical Trial, the child was born blind, with one leg and part of one arm missing, and in Brandt's words "appeared to be an idiot."[25] In that case, the father had written to Hitler "and asked for this child, or this creature, to be put down."[26] From that "small beginning," Hitler launched the "children's euthanasia program," authorizing Brandt and another official, Philipp Bouhler, to deal with similar cases in the same way.[27]

Could it plausibly be argued that this was not a "life worth living," as judged from the infant's point of view? Using Lorber's criterion of an acceptable quality of life, "the ability to work or marry," this child would fall below the line. Is it even possible to make an assessment of the value that child's life could have for him?

Jumping to a recent case, that of Baby Doe born in April 1982 in Bloomington, Indiana, we find that the infant's father did seek to make that assessment for him. Baby Doe was born with a correctable intestinal defect—an improperly formed esophagus. But he was also born with Down's syndrome, the chromosomal anomaly formerly known as mongolism. In the court proceeding that later ensued, the baby's father told the Circuit Court that "he was a schoolteacher and had sometimes worked closely with Down's syndrome children. He said that he and his wife were of the opinion that such children never had a minimally acceptable quality of life."[28] The parents decided that "it was in the best interests of Baby Doe, and also of their family as a whole" to forgo the life-preserving surgery. They understood that although efforts would be made in the hospital to keep the infant comfortable and free of pain, he would die within a short time, either from starvation and dehydration—since he could not be fed by mouth—or from complications leading to pneumonia.[29]

In August 1939, a circular issued by the Reich Interior Ministry mandated a "duty to report deformed births." All newborn infants "suspected of suffering from the following congenital defects" were to be registered: (1) Idiocy and Mongolism (particularly cases that involved blindness and deafness); (2) Microcephalie; (3) Hydrocephalus of a serious or progressive nature; (4) Deformities of every kind, in particular, the absence of limbs, spina bifida, and so on; (5) Paralysis, including Little's disease.[30] Some of these infants were identified by "assessors" (who did not actually examine them) and marked for death. This group was transferred to special "pediatric clinics," where they were either starved to death, given lethal injections, or died of diseases caused by malnutrition.[31]

Thus, some of these children marked for death were actively killed, whereas others were simply allowed to die. Their parents were pressured to allow the infants to be transferred to these special clinics on the grounds that they

would be given "optimum treatment." The stated reason
was an obvious falsehood, clearly intended to deceive the
parents about the purpose of the transfer.[32] Although it was
possible for parents to refuse, they had to sign a declaration
committing themselves to remove the children from the hospital, and provide supervision and care.[33] Again in order to
deceive, the cause of death was listed as "a more or less ordinary disease such as pneumonia, which could even have [a]
kernel of truth...."[34]

The Slippery Slope

This account of the "Children's Euthanasia Program"
brings us to the third, and ultimately the most interesting
approach to comparisons between the Nazi euthanasia program and current practices of withholding or withdrawing
life supports: commentators on the slippery slope. Adherents
of this approach cite the description by Leo Alexander, who
worked with the United States Counsel for War Crimes in
Nuremberg. Alexander wrote that the Nazi euthanasia program

> "started from small beginnings. The beginnings at first
> were merely a subtle shift in emphasis in the basic
> attitude of the physicians...that there is such a thing
> as a life not worthy to be lived. This attitude in its
> early stages concerned itself merely with the severely
> and chronically sick. Gradually the sphere of those to
> be included in this category was enlarged to encom-
> pass the socially unproductive, the ideologically
> unwanted and finally all non-Germans. But it is
> important to realize that the infinitely small wedged-
> in lever from which this entire trend of mind received
> its impetus was the attitude towards the nonrehab-
> ilitable sick."[35]

Assessing the slipperiness of the slope are three camps.
One group contends that there are simply not enough similarities between the Nazis' euthanasia program and today's
practices to cause concern that we have begun the danger-

ous slide down that slope. An example appears in a book by Helga Kuhse and Peter Singer, who write:

"When the Nazis talked of 'a life not worthy to be lived' they meant that the life was unworthy because it did not contribute to the health of that mysterious racial entity, the *Volk*. Since our society does not believe in any such entity, there is no real prospect that allowing active euthanasia of severely handicapped newborn infants would lead to Nazi-style atrocities."[36]

A member of the opposite camp contests that assessment of the likelihood of sliding down the infamous slope. David Lamb writes:

"An immediate reaction to Kuhse and Singer here is that racism in our culture is very much alive and that the homogeneity presupposed by the expression 'our society' simply does not exist. However, it may be the case that despite the existence of racism in Western society, contemporary medicine does not have notions of the 'Volk' at its core. But there is an increasing concern with social utility which may turn out to be not that far removed from the Nazi standpoint."[37]

How far removed a current concern might be from the Nazi standpoint is difficult to determine. Consider a statement made in 1984 by a physician, following the passage of amendments to the Child Abuse and Neglect Prevention and Treatment Act and ensuing federal regulations: "The law now states that in obstetrical units, babies must be fed and given full support regardless of how extensive and hopeless their congenital malformations...These [issues] must be viewed not only in the light of the individual's right to life, but in that of society's right for its members to have pleasant and productive lives, not to be lived mainly to support the growing numbers of hopelessly disabled, often unconscious people whose costly existence is consuming so much of the gross national product..."[38]

The author of this article is careful to point out that he is not referring to defects that can be treated (harelips, spina bifidas, or deformities of the extremities). He does include, however, "totally incurable and accurately diagnosable brain defects" such as Down's syndrome: "No child with Down's syndrome ever grew up to be self-sustaining."

The author is surely not endorsing active euthanasia of Down's syndrome infants or other groups for whom "there should be no reason to support life artificially," such as "old-sters with mental deterioration from stroke or Alzheimer's disease [who have] become totally incompetent to care for themselves..." However, he does assert that "there should be no support from the community or the state" to keep such people alive. It is worth recalling that in 1939, under the children's euthanasia program fashioned by the Nazis, it was possible for parents to refuse to have their children trans-ferred to special "pediatric clinics" if they signed a declara-tion committing themselves to remove the children from the hospital, and provide supervision and care.

Those who are quick to dismiss all attempts to compare the Nazi euthanasia program with current attitudes and prac-tices should reflect soberly on whether society has a "right" for its members to have pleasant and productive lives. The driving force behind the Nazi program was the perception of "growing numbers of hopelessly disabled people who consume so much of the gross national product."

Hitler's adult euthanasia program had a separate orga-nization and history from the children's program. It began with a statement in August, 1939 by Philipp Bouhler, then head of the Party Chancellery, that the purpose of eliminat-ing persons having a "life unworthy of life" was not only to continue the "struggle against genetic disease" but also to free up hospital beds and personnel for the coming war.[39] At a meeting of the "steering group" in October, 1939, this state-ment of purpose was translated into a cost-benefit assess-ment of how many would be killed:

> "The number is arrived at through a calculation on the basis of a ratio of 1000:10:5:1. That means out of 1,000 people 10 require psychiatric treatment; of these

5 in residential form. And, of these, one patient will
come under the programme. If one applies this to the
population of the greater German Reich, then one must
reckon with 65–75,000 cases."[40]

The program proceeded according to schedule, and by
the end of August, 1941, when the gassing phase was ended,
70,273 people had been killed.[41]

The focus of the adult euthanasia program was on adult
chronic patients, especially mental patients. Implementation
of the program involved virtually the entire psychiatric
community, as well as physicians from the general medical
community.[42] In a later phase of the program—referred to
in Nazi documents as "wild euthanasia"—physicians were
empowered to act on their own initiative regrarding who
would live or die.[43]

When the question was posed of how the killings would
be done, the initial answer was again arrived at by a cost-
benefit analysis.

"The number referred to by Party Comrade Brack also
tallies with [Heyde's] own estimation. It makes the
proposed method of injections put forward by Professor Nitsche unviable. For the same reason, the use of
doses of medicine is also impossible...The question has
been discussed with the director of the Reich Criminal Police Department...We are in agreement with
him that CO (Carbon Monoxide) is the best method."[44]

As for just which inmates of psychiatric asylums were
to be selected for the euthanasia program, "the criteria for
assessment were...periodically adjusted."[45] Initially, patients
who could perform useful work were to be excluded from this
action, as well as people who had had a stroke and had
become "mentally defective," and "war disabled who had suffered some kind of mental damage."[46] By 1941, the exclusion
criterion of war service was eliminated.

The final set of criteria for assessment of candidates for
the adult euthanasia program was issued in March, 1941,

before the official ending of the program. The document explicitly excluded senility as a criterion: "Extreme caution in cases of senility. Only urgent cases, e.g., criminals or asocials are to be included...This reference to senile patients does not apply to aged patients with psychoses, such as schizophrenia, epilepsy, etc. who are basically included in the programme."[47] The exclusion of senility as a criterion is interesting in light of the Nazi analogy often invoked when it is suggested today that life prolonging resources be withheld from the elderly based on their chronological age. Not only did the Nazis reject advanced age as a criterion for euthan-asia, but they also urged extreme caution in cases of "ordinary" senility.

Hitler issued a "halt" order in August of 1941, but in practice, it applied only to the large-scale gassing of mental patients. After Hitler's order, the focus shifted to the concentration camps and began to include Jewish prisoners who were neither mentally nor physically sick and thus unable to work. They were selected simply on the basis of race.[48]

A different approach to slippery slope arguments contends that even avowed opponents of that form of argument may have unwittingly begun the slide themselves. Thus, Neuhaus, citing Daniel Callahan's rejection of the Nazi analogy in his discussion of quality of life, observes that Callahan himself has already said:

> "Daniel Callahan is a spirited opponent of the slippery-slope metaphor...but his own emotional preparedness with respect to the treatment of the dependent and incapable has undergone a remarkable development...In...1983...he wrote forcefully against withdrawing food and water...Four years later, Callahan invites us...to discard that moral emotion."[49]

According to Neuhaus, Callahan has slid because to hold that nutrition and hydration may ethically be withheld "requires the erasure of two distinctions of long standing in medical ethics and practice. The first distinction is between 'ordinary' and 'extraordinary' means...and the second distinction is between medical treatment and providing food and water."[50]

Vast literature on the vagueness and ambiguity of the ordinary/extraordinary distinction, and recent work by the President's Commission,[51] seem finally to have laid to rest its utility for the purpose of making ethical judgments. Moreover, one feature of the oft-quoted statement of Pope Pius XII has the potential for being morally pernicious. The 1957 statement holds that "normally one is held to use only ordinary means—means that do not involve any grave burden for oneself or another."[52]

Now what might constitute a grave burden for *another?* A great expenditure of money required to sustain hospitalization and life supports? The agony of a family watching a loved relative linger for months in an intensive care unit? The provision of frequent and unpleasant nursing chores to an incontinent, bedridden, elderly parent with Alzheimer's disease? This feature of the ordinary/extraordinary distinction makes it a criterion for forgoing treatment that is not exclusively patient centered. This opens the door to far wider abuses than abandonment of a distinction found to be unhelpful in medical practice today. To erase the distinction appears to have been a moral gain, rather than a slide down the slope.

Still, it is easy to see how withholding food and water can be assimilated to Nazi practices. The Nazi doctor, Hermann Pfannmuller, was credited with the policy of starving to death those selected for the children's euthanasia program, rather than wasting medication on them.[53] According to the account of a visitor to the institution Pfannmuller directed, he said:

> "We do not kill...with poison, injections, etc.;...No, our method is much simpler and more natural, as you see.'...The murderer explained further then, that sudden withdrawal of food was not employed, rather gradual decrease of the rations. A lady who was also

part of the tour asked—her outrage suppressed with difficulty—whether a quicker death with injections, etc., would not at least be more merciful."[54]

The irony of the visitor's question is a reminder of a core ingredient in the meaning of euthanasia. A lethal injection might very well bring about a more "merciful" death than starvation for these children. But unlike patients in the last throes of terminal illness, the children in the Nazi euthanasia program were deliberately selected to die. It is a cruel irony to voice an ethical indictment of the *mode* of death, when it is the very fact of death that constitutes the moral outrage. The same moral judgment applies to the cases of Baby Doe in Bloomington, Indiana, and the Johns Hopkins baby more than 15 years ago. The fact that they were not fed, and hence starved to death, addresses the lesser of the moral evils. Both infants would have lived if their parents had not refused to consent to surgery to correct their intestinal malformation. And both would have lived had a court order been granted to override parental refusal. There is every reason to believe that these infants suffered.

But there is no reason to believe that irreversibly comatose patients or those in PVS suffer when artificial nutrition and hydration are withheld. These patients have no awareness of their surroundings, nor do they experience sensations. They do not respond to any stimuli, even deep pain. The part of their brain that enables them to have experiences has ceased to function. Therefore, they cannot suffer, either from starvation, dehydration, or continued medical treatment. Whether withdrawal of life supports from such patients should be termed euthanasia is a conceptual question. Whether withdrawal of medical treatment, including artificially administered nutrition and hydration, is ethically acceptable is a separate and distinct question.

There is a third group that remains camped at the base of the slippery slope, watching and waiting. Gregory Pence is prepared to wait and see whether what is for many people the most worrisome practice—active eutha-

nasia, as currently practiced by a few Dutch physicians—
will precipitate the slide:

"What will happen in the future is difficult to predict.
A statute won't solve all problems because it can't be
drafted broadly enough to cover all patients and precisely enough to close loopholes ("terminal condition,"
"unbearable suffering"). In any case, the Dutch experience may show whether mercy killing leads to
Auschwitz, civilized death, or somewhere in between."[55]

Another writer in this camp observes that there's more
than one slope to slide down. Laurence McCullogh argues that
the accuracy of the comparison between the Nazi euthan-asia
program and our own biomedical practices depends on
which features are taken to be relevantly similar or different:

"We see that what got German society on the slippery
slope, indeed what characterized the slope, was the
racist attitudes already in place. It is a reasonable
defence and distinguishes our case from theirs, for us
to say that we don't have those attitudes...*Our* slippery slope might yet be analogous to Germany's in a
more abstract way. If we consider the rationale which
gives social utility or economic returns precedence over
individual freedom, then we might see how our society could approach the kind of thinking that underlay
the Nazi experience. There, racism overrode personal
autonomy; here, it might be an economic rationale—
the attitude that we won't spend so much per year to
keep somebody alive on the slim chance of recovery."[56]

This view is echoed and reinforced by Alan Weisbard
and Mark Siegler, who observe that one slide has already
begun, and now is the time to be vigilant. Their concern is
the acceptance of withholding of food and fluids from dying
patients, conjoined with recent furious efforts to control the
costs of medical care:

"We have witnessed too much history to disregard how
easily society disvalues the lives of the 'unproductive'—

the retarded, the disabled, the senile, the institutionalized, the elderly—of those who in another time and
place were referred to as 'useless eaters.' The
confluence of the emerging stream of medical and ethical opinion favoring legitimation of withholding fluids and nutrition with the torrent of public and
governmental concern over the costs of medical care...
powerfully reinforces our discomfort."[57]

These different worries about the prospect of sliding
down a slippery slope are instructive. Each reveals a somewhat different value bias about euthanasia—what practices
are unacceptable, what we have most to fear, or which of several slopes are most dangerous.

For Neuhaus, it matters not whether euthanasia is
"passive" or "active," "voluntary" or "involuntary." All are
morally wrong. Using the technique known as "persuasive
definition," Neuhaus subsumes all forms of euthanasia under his
broader heading, the "eugenics project."

For Pence, it appears to be both the continued volun-
tariness of the Dutch practice of euthanasia, and its success
in maintaining the limited conditions under which active,
voluntary euthanasia may be performed that would permit
the practice to be ethically acceptable.

For McCullogh, the slide down the slope can be halted
so long as personal autonomy remains paramount, and is not
overridden by economic considerations.

For Callahan, the key lies in paying strict adherence to
an acceptable standard for assessing quality of life. So long
as "borderline cases" are not excluded from the human community, and denied life-preserving therapies on the grounds
that they are lives "not worth living" according to some comparative social standard, we can avoid the murderous tendencies of the Nazi regime.[58]

For Lamb, it is only the ability of our pluralistic society to resist the growing tendencies to violence and increased
tolerance of aggression that can successfully halt a pre-
cipitous slide.[59]

For Weisbard and Siegler, the danger lies in two trends that are reinforcing one another: Monomaniacal concern over the costs of medical care, and acceptance by physicians and society of the ethical acceptability of withholding food and fluids from patients. Weisbard and Siegler state their worries about the slippery slope partly in response to their expressed concern about methods of cost control:

"It may well prove convenient—and all too easy— to move from recognition of an individual's 'right to die'...to a climate enforcing a socially obligatory 'duty to die,' preferably quickly and cheaply."[60]

Concern about still another slippery slope is sometimes voiced about the role physicians are asked to play in voluntary, active euthanasia. If doctors begin to perceive an obligation to kill patients who request it, in addition to their long-standing obligation to heal their patients, they could readily develop an indifference to human beings. Robert Jay Lifton identifies a psychological process he calls "doubling," whereby Nazi doctors could function in their evil role. Lifton describes the process as follows:

"the division of the self into two functioning wholes, so that a part-self acts as an entire self. An Auschwitz doctor could, through doubling, not only kill and contribute to killing but organize silently, on behalf of that evil project, an entire self-structure (or self-process) encompassing virtually all aspects of his behavior."[61]

Whether "doubling," or becoming indifferent to the value of human life, is an inevitable consequence of physicians performing active euthanasia in response to patients' requests is an empirical question, one that can only be answered by observation and experience.

Similarly, a parallel slope envisaging a slide from physicians performing voluntary euthanasia to engaging in involuntary euthanasia requires empirical support. Indeed, some critics of the practice in the Netherlands claim that

already there are numerous instances of involuntary euthanasia, and more will no doubt follow, despite the strict safeguards designed to permit only voluntary euthanasia with
terminally ill patients.

Anyone who tentatively accepts the ethical permissibility of voluntary, active euthanasia would almost certainly
reject its incorporation into social policy if it became evident
that any of these predictions about the slippery slope were
beginning to be realized. Some actions might be morally right
in an ideal world, but should be ruled out in the real world,
given human fallibility and other practical deterrents to at-
taining the ideal.

The Most Dangerous Slope

Critics of today's practices contend that what is afoot is
at least the inception of a programmatic effort to terminate
the lives of some patients. Kronberg refers to the "modern
Euthanasia Movement," claiming that it "is scarcely different from
its Nazi predecessor."[62] Neuhaus refers to "the eugenics
project,"[63] which he takes to include cessation of life-sustaining treatment. More circumspect and less polemical critics,
such as Weisbard and Siegler, assert that the "'death with
dignity' movement has now advanced to a new frontier: the
termination or withdrawal of fluids and nutritional support."[64]

Whether today's medical practices regarding termination
of treatment are referred to as a "project" or "movement," or
described in morally neutral terms, numerous writers remind
us that the Holocaust did not begin with a "euthanasia program." Not only did it start from "small beginnings;" it was
preceded by a period in which resources were scarce, when "there
was a temptation to adopt a narrowly materialistic perspective for the establishment of priorities and to seek savings
through shortcuts at the expense of those who were weak
and less able to defend themselves."[65] It is just such considerations that lead to worries about where we are headed today.

Without specific reference to Nazi practices, that worry is voiced by Leslie Steven Rothenberg, one of the contributors to the Hastings Center's Project on Termination of Treatment Guidelines. Rothenberg writes:

> "The ethical distinction between 'terminating treatment' and 'terminating life' (whether called active euthanasia, mercy killing, assisted suicide, or 'medical killing') may be more important to me than to others, particularly because the health care system is preoccupied with cost containment and because society undervalues persons with disabilities (including those that accompany advanced age)."[66]

For these reasons, Rothenberg dissents from several sections of the *Guidelines*. He expresses the fear that the *Guidelines* "may be used to give a moral 'imprimatur' to undertreating or failing to treat persons with disabilities, unconscious persons for whom accurate prognoses are not yet obtainable, elderly patients with severe dementia, and others whose treatment is not believed...'costworthy.' "[67]

Withholding or withdrawing life-sustaining therapy from patients whose continued treatment is not "costworthy" bears a much greater similarity to the Nazi euthanasia program than does the current practice of active euthanasia in the Netherlands. The "costworthy" rationale also bears a greater similarity to the Nazis' purpose than does the current practice of complying with patients' requests to forgo life supports or following their advance directives regarding medical treatment once they have lost decisional capacity.

A careful reading of the Hastings Center's *Guidelines on the Termination of Life-Sustaining Treatment* reveals a good deal of caution. There is an admonition "to avoid discriminating against the critically ill and dying, to shun invidious comparisons of the economic value of various individuals to society, and to refuse to abandon patients and hasten death to save money."[68] There is a concerted effort in the section entitled "The Use of Economic Considerations in Decisions

Concerning Life-sustaining Treatments" to retain a patient-
centered ethic in medicine.[69]

Yet despite these cautions and concerns, the *Guidelines*
acknowledge the relevance and importance of considerations
of costworthiness. One statement begins with the prohibition: "The health care professional caring for an individual
patient should *not* be involved in cutting costs or rationing
scarce resources at the bedside for the benefit of society," yet
ends with the proviso: "unless it is in accordance with institutional or governmental policy."[70]

This brings us back to the case with which we began—
the family of Holocaust survivors who were unwilling to
reduce the level of care being provided. The patient's physician did not want to be the one to ration resources at the
bedside. There was no institutional policy in place. One ethics committee member questioned whether the hospital ought
to have such a policy, making it easier for physicians to tell
patients or families that an official policy required care to be
withdrawn. The Hastings Center's *Guidelines* state that
"when such policies have been developed according to procedures and standards that are reasonable and just by government or by institutions, it is ethically justifiable for health
care professionals to follow such policies and to refuse to provide this treatment."[71]

In this case, the physician did continue to provide treatment and the patient lived for another seven months, though
she never awakened to recognize her family or interact with
her environment. Despite the pressure exercised by hospital
administration, it is the physicians, not the administration,
who retain final authority in patient management decisions
in that hospital.

Whether it is accurate to call reducing the level of care
for this patient "euthanasia" is not the moral issue. Terminating treatment would not count as 'euthanasia' according
to several of the definitions discussed earlier, but might fit
other definitions. It is ironic to note that on one account, it
would not count as euthanasia but would fit the description
of the Nazi program: "[T]he decision to terminate the life of

a patient under the Nazi programme was taken not by the individual concerned or by his or her relatives but by an official body...[T]he criterion...was not the welfare of the individual patient but whether or not the patient's life was judged to be of 'value' or 'worth'...to the community."[72]

Some find the possibility of allowing active euthanasia—even the voluntary kind—to be the most worrisome prospect. Others fear that from an ethical standpoint, the most dangerous practice is withdrawing or withholding treatment involuntarily, that is, from patients who lack decisional capacity. I maintain that a far greater danger lies in the use of an economic rationale.

When the justification offered for terminating treatment is that it is not "costworthy," or that it is consuming a disproportionate amount of society's or an institution's resources, the slide down one of the slopes to the Nazi program has already started. As one scholar has observed, "the argument for the destruction of life not worth living was at root an economic one."[73]

This is not to overlook the salient fact that racial ideology was a driving force behind Nazi policies. Is our society so free of racism that we are in no danger of sliding down that slope, as well? I think that danger may lurk in the background, but it is likely to arise in an indirect fashion, rather than directly. Although racial prejudice in our society undeniably exists, it does not assume the proportions of an ideology except in the case of fringe sects and fanatic groups. However, since disproportionate numbers of the poor are members of racial or ethnic minorities, a *de facto* pattern of discrimination can be detected.

The pressure to ration health care or to deny access to the health care system to certain members of society is greatest when tax dollars are used to fund services for the poor or indigent. A case in point is refusal by the federal government and a number of states to allow the use of public funds to finance abortions. To the extent that this pattern of health care spending continues, the poor, largely a minority population, are likely to be more negatively affected by schemes to limit the use of life-prolonging measures. Even when government-supported programs pay for all who are in need of a medical treatment, as in the case of end-stage renal disease, it is striking that many more whites receive these life-preserving therapies than do blacks and other minorities.

I do not suggest that efforts cannot be made to halt a slide that has begun. But when a society regularly and systematically confuses economics with ethics, and uses cost-benefit analysis as its only tool in forging health policy, it will fail to recognize the most dangerous slope of all.

From: *When Medicine Went Mad* Ed.: A. Caplan
©1992 The Humana Press Inc.

The Contemporary Euthanasia Movement and the Nazi Euthanasia Program

Are There Meaningful Similarities?

Ronald E. Cranford

In the Netherlands today, it is estimated that as many as 5,000–10,000 patients have their lives ended each year by the practice of active euthanasia (the administration of lethal doses of medications to relieve pain and suffering in the hopelessly ill) by physicians. No one knows the incidence of active euthanasia in the US in the late 1980s, but it is probably not rare, and certainly much more common than in previous decades. Whenever the subject of active euthanasia is debated, the similarities between this practice and the Nazi euthanasia program are raised. This chapter will discuss some of these apparent similarities and differences between the contemporary euthanasia movement and the Nazi euthanasia program of the 1930s and 1940s.

Rational Suicide and Active Euthanasia

In the March 30, 1989, issue of the *New England Journal of Medicine*, I and 11 other physicians in the US published an article on the humane care of the dying entitled

"The Physician's Responsibility Toward The Hopelessly Ill Patient: A Second Look."[1] In this article, we primarily addressed the issue in terms of forgoing life-sustaining treatment and relieving suffering, as we had in our previous article in 1984.[2] We condemned the futile prolongation of life and needless suffering that US physicians too frequently bring about for dying patients. We agreed with the public perception that physicians' attitudes and practices cause a great deal of futile prolongation of life, needless suffering, and loss of control for individuals and families in the dying process. In discussing the dilemma between relieving suffering and killing, we argued strongly that physicians should adequately alleviate suffering, even if there is a remote possibility that the patient will die as a result.

Except for the rather strong criticism of current physician practices, there was nothing new or original in our paper. Our views were similar to positions expressed by other medical/ethical bodies in the recent past, such as the President's Commission for the Study of Ethical Problems in Medicine and the Hastings Center Guidelines on Termination of Treatment and the Care of the Dying.[3,4]

However, we went one step further. In discussing suicide and rational suicide, we said that in rare circumstances, it is not immoral for a physician to assist in the rational suicide of a terminally ill patient. We stressed that this should be a rare situation, but we did break new ground in taking this controversial position.

Even though the issue of active euthanasia was extensively discussed, there was no consensus whatsoever among the physicians, and we took no definitive position in this area except to describe the current scene. Recognizing major medical, moral, and legal distinctions between killing and allowing to die, and that in most circumstances there is a well-demarcated line between the two, we nevertheless crossed the line and condoned a form of killing.

Why did we do this? Why did we take this somewhat radical step? First and foremost, we did this because we believed it. We felt that there are situations (granted, they are rare) where it is moral for a physician to assist a patient in a rational suicide. We had reached a consensus that there is such a thing as rational suicide. AIDS, for example, has forced us to change our thinking on many medicine and public health issues; one of them is the question of rational suicide. Unfortunately, some of the overwhelming suffering that AIDS patients endure in the final stages of this disease can only be relieved by suicide. Our paper stressed, however, that if there were more humane care of the dying in allowing to die situations, there would be much less pressure toward suicide and active euthanasia.

There were two other reasons why we took this step. In 1988, four distinguished national medical ethicists—Drs. Siegler, Kass, Pellegrino, and Gaylin—published an editorial in the *Journal of the American Medical Association*.[5] They expressed their views in response to the "Debbie" episode, in which a physician admitted that he had committed active euthanasia on a young female patient who was apparently suffering from intolerable pain with end-stage cancer.[6] After this admission, debates ranged from the way the physician committed active euthanasia to whether he had performed active euthanasia at all.[7-9] In their editorial, these medical ethicists not only deplored the actions of this physician, but also strongly insisted that there should be no debate whatsoever on the merits of active euthanasia and that this "outrageous" practice, like "incest and slavery," should not be discussed by "decent folk." We wanted to disagree with their position. Active euthanasia and physician-assisted suicide are occurring in the US, and it is no longer an issue that can simply be ignored. Whatever one's views on the merits of physician-assisted suicide and active euthanasia, we felt the issue should be debated. So, one major reason for publishing our views on physician-assisted suicide was the same as a major reason for this conference: to debate an extremely controversial topic that needs to be debated. The other reason for publishing our views was because of our concern about the great amount of hypocrisy, deception, and denial of reality characteristic of many physicians in the US today. Physicians (and others) argue that the Oath of Hippocrates contains an absolute prohibition against killing (a view with substantial merit), but these same physicians, in our opinion, cause a great deal of suffering through their inadequate treatment of pain and other distressing symptoms that occur during the dying process. These very physicians, so violently opposed to active euthanasia because they feel it is a violation of the Oath of Hippocrates, can be seen as violating the Oath in another way: by causing needless suffering. We felt that such an unacceptable practice indicates considerable professional hypocrisy. In fact, the two groups most opposed to active euthanasia in the US and in the world today are the two groups that, I feel, will most likely facilitate the movement toward active euthanasia. These are the medical profession and the pro-life groups. By presenting the greatest obstacles to developing policies on the humane care toward the dying, these two groups augment the grassroots pressure toward suicide and active euthanasia.

The Contemporary Euthanasia Movement and the Nazi Euthanasia Program

Since euthanasia is a topic in current medical practice, we might do well to consider the similarities and differences between the Nazi euthanasia program of 1933–1945 and the contemporary euthanasia movement in the US and the world. There are, as one might expect, radical differences between the two.

First, from the earliest stages, the Nazi euthanasia program was never intended to benefit the individual. The program was always intended to further the objectives and goals of the "volk," a term that in the abstract means "nation" or "people," but, as the Nazis used it, meant the German Aryan people whom they regarded as inherently superior. Nazi programs were always intended to further the goal of Aryan supremacy, even from the very beginning. Second, the program was never voluntary. Not only was consent never obtained from the hapless victims, but they would have never given consent had they known what was going to be done to them. Third, the program was never really intended as mercy or compassion for the individual patient who was suffering. The pretense of the Nazi party—that this program was undertaken for the relief of suffering of the individual as a humanitarian, compassionate measure—was a complete propaganda sham from beginning to end.[10,11]

In contrast, the contemporary euthanasia movement is, first and foremost, founded on respect for the autonomy of the individual, not on some abstract social goal. Second, the contemporary movement is for the benefit of the individual and is based on the voluntary consent of the patient. Third, it is intended to relieve the suffering of the individual (mercy killing).[12,13]

Furthermore, the dilemma of the contemporary euthanasia program is the opposite of the dilemma of the Nazi program. The contemporary euthanasia movement centers on the needs and rights of the individual and holds that the individual's right to make decisions concerning his or her own life, including the right to end it, takes precedence over social interests and needs. The critical question is: What adverse implications or impact does this have on broad social values, such as respect for the sanctity of life in general and the potential abuse or discrimination against disadvantaged patients?

In the Nazi euthanasia program, on the other hand, the driving force was furtherance of the volk. Social values prevailed over individual values and the dignity of the individual person. The Nazi program did not lead simply to the abuse of individual patients, but to the most heinous medical moral crimes of the 20th century.

The Dutch Experience

The Netherlands is the only country in the world where the practice of active euthanasia is widely accepted and practiced. My feeling is that the commonly quoted figure of 5,000–10,000 patients dying each year of active euthanasia is probably too high, but no one knows with any degree of certainty. Whereas active euthanasia is not legal in the sense that the Dutch Parliament has specifically legalized it, nevertheless, the practice has been widely accepted by repeated court decisions in the Netherlands, and is also endorsed by the Dutch Medical Association and a governmental commission on euthanasia.[14–16] The Dutch Medical Association emphasizes that active euthanasia should be done only by a physician. The Dutch physicians are adamant that active euthanasia should only be done with the consent of the patient. There are numerous informal criteria or standards for the practice of active euthanasia in the Netherlands, but the most commonly used are the Rotterdam criteria, named for a decision before one court in the Netherlands. The five major features of these Rotterdam criteria are:

1. The patient must be competent and the request voluntary.
2. The request must be repeated and be very clear.
3. There must be intolerable suffering and no alternative treatments to alleviate this suffering.
4. Euthanasia must be done only by a physician.
5. A second physician, one experienced in this practice, should be involved.[17]

When I first learned about the practice of euthanasia in the Netherlands, one of the things that most impressed me was that active euthanasia was performed within the context of a close patient/physician relationship; often, patients had known their general practitioner for 10 or 20 years. Furthermore, unlike in the US, this practice did not entail any legal or economic ramifications. There are no major medical malpractice problems in the Netherlands, nor are there any major economic considerations regarding active euthanasia. The Dutch physicians emphasize that active euthanasia should only be done on competent patients and feel that the United States' practice of stopping treatment on incompetent patients without their consent and perhaps for economic reasons is far more dangerous than euthanasia as practiced in the Netherlands.

The Netherlands is one of the most open societies in the world; medical practices and other social activities are usually not done in a secretive fashion. Furthermore, it is said that the Netherlands has one of the most liberal abortion laws in the world and yet one of the lowest rates of abortion. But the social, economic, political, and legal conditions in the Netherlands are so different from those in the US that one cannot extrapolate from the Dutch practice of active euthanasia and make any definitive recommendations regarding this practice in the US.

The Dutch Resistance During the Nazi Occupation

In contrast to the widespread acceptance of active euthanasia in the Netherlands and the endorsement of this practice by the Dutch medical profession today, the Dutch physicians were the only physicians in any of the occupied European countries of Nazi Germany that resisted the Nazi euthanasia program during World War II. This telling point dramatically emphasizes the radical differences between the Nazi euthanasia program and the contemporary euthanasia movement.

In 1949, Leo Alexander published an article in the *New England Journal of Medicine* entitled "Medical Science Under Dictatorship."[18] In this article, he discussed the example of successful resistance by the physicians of the Netherlands.

> There is no doubt that in Germany itself, the first and foremost effective step of propaganda within the medical professional was the propaganda barrage against the useless, incurably sick described above. Similar, even more subtle efforts were made in some of the occupied countries. It is to the everlasting honor of the medical profession of Holland that they recognized the earliest and most subtle phases of this attempt and rejected it. When Seiss-Inquart, Reich Commis-

sar for the Occupied Netherlands Territories, wanted
to draw the Dutch physicians into the orbit of the
activities of the German medical profession, he did
not tell them 'you must send your chronic patients to
death factories' or 'you must give lethal injections at
government request in your offices,' but he couched
his order in the most careful and superficially acceptable terms. One of the paragraphs in the order of the
Reich Commissar of the Netherlands Territories concerning the Netherlands doctors of 19 December 1941
reads as follows:

> "It is the duty of the doctor, through advice
> and effort, conscientiously and to his best abil-
> ity, to assist as helper to the person entrusted
> to his care in the maintenance, improvement,
> and re-establishment of his vitality, physical
> efficiency and health. The accomplishment of
> this duty is a public task."

Alexander continues:

> The physicians of Holland rejected this or-
> der unanimously because they saw what it
> actually meant—namely the concentration
> of their efforts on mere rehabilitation of the
> sick for useful labor, and abolishment of
> medical secrecy. Although on the surface, the
> order appeared not too grossly unacceptable,
> the Dutch physicians decided that it was the
> first, although slight, step away from prin-
> ciple that is the most important one. The
> Dutch physicians declared that they would
> not obey this order. When Seiss-Inquart
> threatened them with revocation of their
> licenses, they returned their licenses, removed
> their shingles, and while seeing their own
> patients secretly, no longer wrote birth or
> death certificates. Seiss-Inquart retraced
> his steps and tried to cajole them—still to

no effect. Then he arrested 100 Dutch physicians and sent them to concentration
camps. The medical profession remained
adamant and quietly took care of their widows
and orphans, but would not give in. Thus, it
came about that not a single euthanasia or
non-therapeutic sterilization was recommended or participated in by any Dutch physician. They had the foresight to resist before
the first step was taken, and they acted
unanimously and won out in the end. It is
obvious that, if the medical profession of a
small nation under a conqueror's shield could
resist so effectively, the German medical profession could likewise have resisted had they
not taken the fatal first step. It is the first
seemingly innocent step away from principle
that frequently decides a career of crime.
Corrosion begins in microscopic proportions."[18]

Conclusion

One should not interpret my comments as indicating
support for the contemporary euthanasia movement, nor for
the Dutch experience. I simply want to make the point, in
the strongest possible language, that it is an insult to thinking people to suggest that there are meaningful analogies
between the contemporary euthanasia movement and the
Nazi euthanasia program.

We learn from the past. We know that the Nazi euthanasia
program and the Holocaust were purely evil. But the critical
question remains. Was their behavior aberrant in kind or
degree? That is the most critical question before this conference.

Could it happen again? Do we contain the seeds of
Nazism ourselves? I believe the Nazi aberration was one of
degree, not one of kind. The Nazis did not display a different
kind of inhumanity, but rather a *degree* of inhumanity

unparalleled in the annals of human civilization. In contemporary society, there are numerous instances of great hypocrisy, deception, and denial of reality that contain the kernels of abuse that could give rise to at least some of the abuses seen under the Nazi system. We must guard against them.[19]

From: *When Medicine Went Mad* Ed.: A. Caplan
©1992 The Humana Press Inc.

The Way They Were, The Way We Are

Richard John Neuhaus

My assigned topic is "the use of metaphors and analogies concerning the Holocaust in contemporary bioethical debates." The very statement of the topic reflects a high estimate of the human capacity for reasonable discourse. In the view of many, any suggestion that there may be analogies between the way the Nazis were and the way we are, between what they did and what we are doing and proposing to do, is simply intolerable. The very suspicion of such similarities is too painful to bear. As Eliot observes in *Murder in the Cathedral*, "Human kind cannot bear very much reality."

Reasonable discourse requires a measure of dispassion, a critical distancing of ourselves from our emotions, intentions, and interests. This is not easy for any of us, and the higher the stakes the more strongly are our defensive resources engaged. The stakes in the debates under discussion are very high indeed: Who shall live? Who shall die? Who does and who does not belong to the community for which we accept common responsibility? Most of us want to defend most particularly our intentions, our inward dispositions. We may acknowledge that we make mistakes, even that we have done the wrong thing, but we adamantly insist that we meant to do good. If we do not exercise care, reasonable discourse about right and wrong can easily be swamped by the language of intentionality.

Please note that in this chapter I am using the term "Holocaust" inclusively in order to cover the constellation of crimes against humanity that we associate with the Third Reich. Of course the term is often used to refer only to the genocide against the Jews. But in that limited sense the Holocaust has little relevance to bioethical debates today. Nobody of influence in our society is proposing the elimination of Jews. Nor did the Nazis one day decide it would be a great idea to kill six million Jews and millions of other "subhuman" human beings. The way to crimes against humanity was prepared by peculiar ways of thinking about humanity. As Richard Weaver insisted, "Ideas have consequences." The Holocaust was, in largest part, the consequence of ideas about human nature, human rights, the imperatives of history and scientific progress, the character of law, the bonds and obligations of political community. It is above all in the exploration of ideas that we can most usefully discuss the "metaphors and analogies" between then and now.

Please note also—and this I want to say most emphatically—the present chapter is an exploration and not an accusation. I make no claim to being "value-neutral" with respect to the subject at hand. I hope that nobody here makes that claim. The purpose is to examine the value judgments and moral reasoning that inform current debates and practices, and to reflect on their similarities and dissimilarities with the Holocaust. If I suggest that a certain line of reasoning is disturbingly reminiscent of the Holocaust, I am not suggesting that those who think that way are morally equivalent to the perpetrators of the Holocaust. The stipulation throughout is that all the participants in current debates intend to do good and not evil. One may morally challenge practices as various as abortion, embryo experimentation, fetal transplants, assisted suicide, and active euthanasia, and, at the same time, acknowledge that there are important distinctions to be made among these practices, distinctions that make a moral difference.

The focus here is on ideas and their use as justifying rationales for doing this or that. The debates will continue and, if they are to be both civil and clarifying debates, it is important that we not impugn the motives of those with whom we disagree. Intentions are not everything, but neither are they nothing. The present examination is for each of us also a self-examination. It assumes that, as we believe ourselves to be capable of great good, we know we are also capable of great evil, our intentions notwithstanding. If that assumption is not shared, this conference is, in the dismissive sense of the term, no more than an academic exercise. If we know in advance that we could not and will not commit crimes against humanity, the question posed by this conference has already been answered and we might as well adjourn the meeting.

One kind of reaction to the question posed is described by two participants in the National Institutes of Health panel on fetal transplantation. Their minority report observes, "Another vindication of fetal research with aborted tissue was grounded on the assumption that our inward dispositions alone determine the ethical value of our behavior. Several senior research sponsors expressed to the Panel their indignation that the work to which they had dedicated years of good will could be considered exploitative. They resented having their integrity appraised by reference to anything but their good intentions." As we shall see, this very insistence on the sufficiency of intention has its counterpart in the experience of the Holocaust.

I do not wish to get into the linguistic technicalities of what is meant by "metaphor" or "analogy" or other literary tropes. Our subject is the way they were and the way we are, what they did and what we are doing and proposing to do. The question is one of likenesses and unlikenesses, of similarities and dissimilarities between then and now. And a prior question, that cannot be ignored, is about the very legitimacy of inquiring into comparisons between the Holocaust and present developments in bioethics. The very calling of this conference assumes that that prior question has been answered, and I believe it has been answered correctly. It is not only legitimate, it is morally imperative that all of us who live after the Holocaust examine ourselves and our actions by reference to that moment of awesome truth.

The invocation of the Holocaust must be undertaken with most particular caution and clarity. For those of us in the West, the Holocaust is probably the only culturally available icon of absolute evil. Any "revisionist" efforts to deny or diminish the horror of the Holocaust are, quite rightly, deemed to be beyond the pale of responsible discourse. It is not only the so-called revisionists, however, who distort the Holocaust and its continuing pertinence. There are those who insist on the uniqueness, the utter singularity of the Holo- caust in a manner that consigns it to the unusable past. If the Holocaust is like nothing else, it is relevant to nothing else.

As we must attend to similarities between then and now, we must also attend to dissimilarities. There are dangers in universalizing or generalizing the Holocaust in ways that obscure the historical particularity of the event and that obscure, as well, the particular ideas, decisions, actions, and attitudes that are the parts that make up the whole of what we call the Holocaust. We intend to honor the victims when we speak of the "six million" or the "10 million," but both killed and killers should, as much as possible, be recalled by name, for they had names. The Holocaust was not the abstraction we call a period of history but a succession of mornings and afternoons and evenings, much like this day. It was a tangled combination of innumerable actions and con- sequences, of careers and ambitions, of fears and loyalties, of flirtations with the unthinkable turning into the routines of the unexceptionable. To most of those involved, the icon of evil did not present itself whole. It happened an hour at a time, an equivocation at a time, a lie at a time, a decision at a time, a decision evaded at a time. There is great wisdom in Hannah Arendt's description of the Holocaust in terms of "the banality of evil."

A generalized Holocaust is deprived of its power to cau- tion and instruct. A generalized Holocaust is a depersonalized Holocaust, replacing persons with statistics, with allegedly inexorable forces of history. Raskolnikov, the murderer in

Crime and Punishment, well understood the uses of generalization. "Anyway, to hell with it! Let them [die]! That's how it should be, they say. It's essential, they say, that such a percentage should every year go—that way—to the devil—it's essential so that the others should be kept fresh and healthy and not be interfered with. A percentage! What fine words they use, to be sure! So soothing. Scientific. All you have to do is say 'percentage' and all your worries are over. Now, of course, if you used some other word—well, then perhaps it would make you feel a little uncomfortable."

This meeting would be a failure were we not made to feel uncomfortable. The more subtle truth is that it would be an even greater failure were we made to feel more comfortable because we feel uncomfortable. Our discomfort testifies to our moral integrity, or so we like to think. The suspicion is not entirely unwarranted that the relatively new profession of bioethics was established to cater to our discomfort and thus to relieve our discomfort. There are things we would not do without professional permission; what is morally doubtful must be certified by expertly guided anguish. In connection with so many life and death questions today, we hear much talk about difficult and anguishing decisions. Anguish, some seem to believe, covers a multitude of sins. In pondering analogies with the Holocaust, we may be inclined to think that this is what distinguishes us from them: We know what we are doing, we recognize and openly discuss the potential risks and potential wrongs, and our decisions are accompanied by the prescribed quota of anguish.

Please do not misunderstand. The emergence of the profession of bioethics does testify to our culture's moral sensitivity. Maybe the profession has prevented and will prevent moral enormities that might otherwise be perpetrated. Maybe. With respect to what was not thought before, or with respect to what was thought and thought to be unthinkable before, bioethics may be producing more preventions than permissions. I do not know, and I do not know if such a calculation is even possible. Would developments similar to those of the Holocaust be better kept at bay were there no discipline called bioethics? That is eminently debatable. Is professional bioethics in any sense an independent variable, so to speak, or simply the mistress of the "hard" disciplines it is employed to serve? Again, I do not know, although I know and am encouraged by the fact that there are those in the field who are not indifferent to these questions about their work.

I am reliably informed that the most typical Jewish telegram reads: "Start worrying. Letter to follow." One does not have to be Jewish to recognize that worry and anguish can be signs of health. With respect to current and proposed medical and biological practices, the letter is arriving page by page and we know that there is a good deal to worry about. It is easy to be alarmist; it is easier to deny that there is cause for alarm. I am convinced that there are unmistakable similarities between what they did then and what we are doing now. They too asked and answered the question, Who shall live and who shall die? And, Who belongs to the community entitled to our protection? Then and now, the subject at hand is killing, and letting die, and helping to die, and using the dead. Then and now, the goal is to produce healthier human beings and, perhaps, a better quality of human being.

It will not do to say that the difference is that our intentions are good whereas theirs were evil. Neither will it do to say that they were cruel and callous whereas we are sensitive and professionally tutored in the arts of anguish. Appealing to good intentions and producing the requisite quota of anguish are question-begging responses to the problems posed. Good intentions and delicate sensibilities are not moral arguments. Anyone familiar with the literature of the Holocaust knows all too well how its perpetrators invoked good intentions and evidences of moral sensitivity to justify their actions, both during and after the fact. We are inclined to dismiss such appeals as smarmy sentimentality and self-serving rationalization, and understandably so. But it is not always sufficiently clear on what grounds we so easily dismiss their justifications, thus, denying any similarity between them and us. Sometimes we seem to be saying that we are not like them because we are not like them. If we are satisfied with that tautology, it would seem that this conference and similar explorations are a waste of time. Obviously, that tautology does not satisfy us, or we would not be here.

All of us are joined in declaring "Never Again!" It would make no sense to say "Never Again!" unless we believed that it could happen again. With the motto "Never Again!" we aim to stir our society from the smug and irrational confidence that it cannot happen here. Of course then is not now, and there is not here, and they are not us. If or when it happens again, we will, to paraphrase the popular song, do it our way. Since those who do it may continue to be in charge, since there may never be the equivalent of the Nuremberg trials, it will be called not Holocaust but Progress. We need never fear the charge of crimes against humanity so long as we hold the power to define who does and who does not belong to "humanity." Is entertaining the possibility that "it" could happen again alarmist? I think not. It is undoubtedly alarming. To be alarmed is a sign of moral sanity.

Emil Fackenheim has wisely said, "We must grant Hitler no posthumous victories." It would seem to follow that we must not grant Hitler the posthumous victory of hiding from ourselves what we are capable of doing, what we may already be doing. Elie Wiesel has written, "If we forget, we are guilty, we are accomplices... I swore never to be silent whenever and wherever human beings endure suffering and humiliation. We must always take sides. Neutrality helps the oppressor, never the victim." The use of the first person plural "we," underscores the fact of moral agency and moral responsibility. The Holocaust began in depersonalizing the victims and ended in depersonalizing the perpetrators. The decisions and actions that we are discussing here are not undertaken by the "logic of history," nor by "medical science," nor by "technological progress," nor by "the imperatives of research." They are undertaken by us, the first person plural composed of first persons singular. Moral agents have names. To seek escape in anonymity, to blame forces beyond our control for decisions within our control is already to have granted Hitler a posthumous victory.

Samuel and Pearl Oliner recently published a book that, in my judgment, has not received the attention it deserves. *The Altruistic Personality* is based on in-depth interviews with hundreds of people who, at great risk to their own lives and the lives of their family, rescued Jews from the Holocaust. The Oliners ask what distinguished the rescuers from the overwhelming majority of people who averted their gaze from what was happening, or were actively complicit in what afterward were called crimes against humanity. Their conclusion is that the rescuers were distinguished not by their educational level, nor by their political views, nor by any other number of variables that might be supposed. They were not even distinguished by their attitudes toward Jews as such.

They were different in two critical respects. They typically had strong ties to communities that espoused rather straightforward and unsophisticated understandings of right and wrong. And they uniformly had an unquenchable sense of personal moral agency. One after another, they told the Oliners that they could not have lived with themselves—and, many added, they could not have answered to God—if they had not done what they had done.

They had been told that what was happening was not their responsibility, that an entirely new situation demanded anguishing decisions that could no longer be avoided, that scientific and historical necessity required a rethinking of familiar values, that traditional views had to give way to the inexorable course of progress, that short-term sacrifices of customary ways was the price of long-term advancement, and that, in any event, people wiser than themselves had thought these things through with great care, and who were they to challenge the experts and those in authority? All this they were told, and all this they refused to believe. They refused to surrender their knowledge of moral agency. As many would still say today, they refused to surrender their souls. They refused to grant Hitler that victory.

In the debate over abortion there has been much discussion surrounding "the seamless garment" as a metaphor for the so-called "life issues." I will not here enter into that debate within a debate, except to note that evil, like good, does seem to weave a pattern. We are considering here the finished pattern, the "final solution," that we call the Holocaust. The finished product may not be seamless; there are disruptions and disjunctions here and there, but the end result is of a piece. And so it is with current debates in bioethics. Consider, for instance, the NIH panel on fetal transplation. The majority report is touchingly eager in its insistence that fetal transplation should and can be separated from the question of abortion. Commenting on the statement of Elie Wiesel cited above, the minority report says: "Wiesel is saying that even by acquiescent silence after the fact we can sign on as parties to a deed already done. But what we are considering here is no mere post-mortem silence, no simple averting of the gaze after the fact. We are considering an institutional partnership, federally sponsored and financed, whereby the bodily remains of abortion victims become a regularly supplied medical commodity."[1]

The minority makes a convincing case, I believe, that the majority deludes itself if it really thinks that the question of fetal transplants can be isolated from the question of how the fetuses are obtained. The minority report, written by James Bopp and James Burtchaell, points out that fetal transplation would almost certainly increase the number of abortions, compound the collusion between medical healing and medicalized killing, and prepare the way for other steps that would not only parallel but replicate actions associated with the Holocaust. In an important sense, this minority report is saying nothing new. Dr. Johnson famously observed that mankind needs less to be instructed than to be reminded. In this instance, we need to be reminded of the War Crimes Trial in Nuremberg known as "The Medical Case."

That trial produced the Nuremberg Code of 1946 that began to provide protection for human subjects of research and inspired, in due course, the Declarations of Helsinki in 1964 and 1975. The minority report observes, "Without Nuremberg and its judgment the world's conscience might never have gazed head-on at the intrinsic depravity of the

doctor's defense... The insight of Nuremberg taught us that
when we take possession of others, when their bodies are forc-
ibly delivered up to be used as we wish, then no antecedent
good will and no subsequent scientific yield will absolve us
from having been confederates in their oppression... The Nazi
doctors had learned the ethic of their profession: That a physician may not relieve one human being's affliction at the
cost of another fellow human's suffering. But they contrived
to believe that if an associate had already done the subjugat-
ing and they then did the healing-oriented research, they
could divide the responsibility down the middle. The Tribunal and the world judged otherwise—and condemned the
researchers for it all."

The chief defendant at Nuremberg, the notorious Dr.
Karl Brandt, had once hoped to join Dr. Albert Schweitzer in
his humanitarian work in Africa. Brandt testified to the court
of his great anguish in having to do things in the "interests of
the community" when confronted by the "hard necessity" of
finding ways to protect the population against death and epidemics. Toward that end, the State, the "law of the land,"
gave him permission to experiment on human subjects put
at his disposal. Brandt declared, "There is no prohibition
against daring to progress."

We should not avoid asking ourselves the painfully
obvious question: Do we now think that the judgment at
Nuremberg was in error? Was the 'doctor's defense' right
after all? Should the Dr. Brandts of the Holocaust have been
acquitted? There are many today who seem to be answering
those questions in the affirmative, at least by implication.
More commonly, they condemn what the doctors did then
while approving what the doctors do now, without addressing
the differences between then and now in principle, actual
practice, or justifying rationale. When challenged on the similarities between then and now, many of our contemporaries
are reflexively offended by the suggestion that such a comparison might even be thought worthy of consideration. Such
indignation is frequently followed by taking refuge in the tautology that we are not like them because we are not like them.

A rabbinical dictum has it that we should "place fences around the law." The idea is that restraints and prohibitions should be in place to prevent us from reaching, or at least impede our progress toward, the point of absolute and damning transgression. There should at least be safety rails around the abyss. Perhaps the best that our culture can provide are signposts warning against the danger ahead. The judgment at Nuremberg was such a signpost. It is no longer secure. Perhaps the signpost has been taken down. The Hippocratic Oath was another such signpost. It was. Leon Kass of the University of Chicago has written persuasively about the ominous implications in current revisions and, in effect, rejections of the Hippocratic Oath. When the fences and the safety rails have been removed, when the signposts have been changed or taken down, what reason is there to believe that people in our time will not do what was done then? Such confidence, it is to be feared, is based on little more than sentimental naivete and the unseemly *hubris* of our assumed moral superiority to "them."

But now, it may be objected, the introduction of the issue of fetal transplants and its connection with abortion has turned the discussion toward a subject that we wanted to avoid, abortion. Alternatively, it is said that the important debates in bioethics must move "beyond" the question of abortion. The abortion debate is weary, and we have no doubt all been wearied by it. What that is new could possibly be said in the abortion debate? Perhaps nothing. But again we are reminded of Dr. Johnson's axiom that we have more need to be reminded than to be instructed—or than to be engaged by "new insights." Whether by inherent logic or by historical accident, almost every controverted question in bioethics is entangled with the question of abortion. Again and again, we discover that we cannot go around, but must again go through the abortion debate. Before us are questions about who shall live and who shall die; questions about killing, letting die, helping to die, and using the dead; questions about what or who belongs to the community of legal protection—and when a "what" becomes a "who," and when, at the end of life, a "who" becomes a "what."

Even if some of the great questions that occupy bioethics might theoretically be isolated from the question of abortion, they seldom can be in cultural and political fact. Whether by inherent logic or by historical accident, the abortion debate has become the magnet to which all the other life-and-death debates are attached. We can try to pull them away from that debate, but they are inexorably drawn back to it. Leaving aside for the moment the pro-choice arguments in favor of the abortion liberty, it seems clear that great science-based industries, trajectories of medical experimentation, and perhaps the profession of bioethics itself rest in large part on the settlement articulated in *Roe v. Wade* and related decisions. It seems equally clear that that settlement is by no means settled, and "the law of the land" may in the foreseeable future give way to the laws of 50 states. In ways even more relentless and entangled than at present, arguments about what we insist are "other" questions will be emerging from and returning to the question of abortion. A measure of moral clarity and societal consensus can only be achieved on the far side of the abortion debate, and that far side is not yet within sight.

Those who support the abortion liberty are understandably outraged when their opponents compare the more than 20 million abortions since *Roe v. Wade* with the Holocaust. And it must be noted that the Holocaust is often invoked recklessly and unfeelingly, as though it were simply another convenient stick with which to beat the opposition. In such cases, the only culturally available icon of absolute evil—a precious thing for any culture to possess—is dangerously debased. At the same time, however, we must ask: *If* one believes that 20 million abortions are equivalent to 20 million instances of the taking of innocent human life, does not the analogy with the Holocaust become more appropriate? Perhaps even inevitable? The cultural and political reality is that millions of Americans, a majority of Americans, believe that abortion is precisely that—the taking of an innocent human life. The same Americans are not in agreement on what that perception of reality should mean in terms of abortion law but, if we believe in a society governed by democratic discourse and decision, that perception of reality and the consideration of its legal ramifications cannot be ruled out of order.

One of the lawyers who prosecuted the Nazis in the war crimes trials explained how people could have acted so savagely: "There is only one step to take. You may not think it possible to take it; but I assure you that men I thought decent men did take it. You have only to decide that one group of human beings have lost human rights." But, the objection is heard, such an observation is irrelevant to our discussion of bioethics and the Holocaust. In abortion, in fetal transplants, in embryo experimentation, in new methods of fertilization, in withdrawing food and water from the comatose—in all these instances, we may want to object, we are not dealing with "human beings." But we must ask whether such an objection is not touchingly naive. It assumes one favored outcome of the debate that is still underway over who or what is a human being. It will not do to employ the fatuous rhetorical device of declaring that the other party must be wrong because I am right.

"There is only one step to take," the prosecutor said. In the case of the debates in which we are now embroiled, I suspect that step was in the adoption of the idea of "quality of life" as an indicator of who is and who is not to count as a human being. Then they spoke of *lebensunwertes Leben*, life that is unworthy of life. It is by no means clear to many thoughtful people how we, in principle or in practice, distinguish *lebensunwertes Leben* from a "quality of life index." But, we insist, it should be clear. After all, in the Holocaust they were killing actual human beings, people who were undeniably, not just potentially or marginally, *real people with real rights*. But, once again, it seems that we are found to be begging the question. It is exactly the point that they *did* deny what we take to be undeniable. Similarly, with respect to such issues as abortion, fetal experimentation, and euthanasia, many today deny what an earlier generation and, it would seem, most Americans today take to be undeniable.

That Jews, gypsies, homosexuals, Slavs, and others were not human beings in the full meaning of the term *(Roe v. Wade)* was the doctrine of the Third Reich. Such people were clearly not included in the community of legal rights, protections, and entitlements. Such was the law of the land; such was the view of those who were declared to be "the best and the brightest" of that society. Who was to say that they were wrong? A relatively few daring souls, such as Pastor Dietrich Bonhoeffer, said they were wrong, and paid with their lives. They said the Nazis were wrong on the basis of clear reason, civilizational tradition (remember the fences and signposts), and biblical faith.

And the rescuers studied by the Oliners said they were wrong, and acted courageously on that conviction. Some of them explained their actions in terms similar to those articulated by the Bonhoeffers. Many others, it seems, acted because that is the way they had been taught to act, they could not act differently and still be themselves. Others seemed to have acted instinctively, intuitively. They had, one might say, a nose for evil. They were a small minority, acting outside the law and against the law, in a society that acknowledged no law other than the fiat of the State. It requires no great leap of creative imagination to see the parallels, at least with respect to their social placement and psychology, between the rescuers then and efforts such as Operation Rescue now.

I have written elsewhere about what I believe is accurately described as "the return of eugenics." By that phrase I mean to include most of the controverted issues in bioethics—from fetal farming and harvesting to infanticide and assisted suicide. We tell ourselves that these issues are raised by medical and technological advances, and so we seek to reduce our sense of moral agency and responsibility. We are closer to the truth, I believe, if we acknowledge that the debates in which we are embroiled are the products of moral, cultural, and political change. Christopher Lasch has recently and insightfully written about "the engineering of the good life." He notes that there are no longer freak shows at carnivals and county fairs. The reason for that, we tell ourselves, is that as a society we have become more sensitive to the handicapped, or, as we are tutored to say, "the differently advantaged." Lasch suggests that this may be a convenient self-deception. The reason there are no more freak shows, he suggests, is that we have become a society that has no place for freaks.

At Nuremberg the prosecution argued that the killing programs unfolded from one another, that the genocide of the six millionth Jew was somehow unleashed by the morphine overdose given to the first harelipped child. Judgment at Nuremberg was premised on the now frequently derided notion of the slippery slope. Those who deride and dismiss that metaphor are, I believe, rejecting the commonsensical observation that one thing is connected with another, and one thing frequently leads to another. If we give ourselves permission to do one thing, we are inescapably inviting the question about permission to do the next thing. Most current debates in bioethics have less to do with technological progress than with moral permissions. In largest part, the profession of bioethics is the Permissions Office of contemporary medical and biological science. Bioethicists are permitted to give out permission slips, with the understanding that, after due and anguished deliberation, permission will not be refused. It is the bold bioethicist who dares to say, and continues to say, No. As he or she may quickly discover, the profession leaves such sensitive souls behind as the discussion moves on to the next thing.

It is easy to be alarmist; it is easier to deny the reason for alarm. We say we know the difference between questionable human life and undeniable human life, while it is evident to all but the willfully blind that lives once thought to be undeniably human are now thrown into question. Again, the awesome step was taken with *Roe v. Wade*. In the lethal illogic of that decision, it might be suggested, we encountered our first harelipped child. The late Paul Ramsey tirelessly reminded us that we should not give ourselves a principle of permission to do what we want if the same principle permits the doing of what we abhor. A principle established by the scrupulous is no longer the exclusive property of the scrupulous. It is public and it is entrenched in practice, there to be exploited by others who view our abhorrence as no more than irrational inconsistency.

We think of the Holocaust as a rampage of irrationality, but as we tend to overlook the banality of evil so also we overlook the rationality of evil. Consider a recent and acclaimed work in this area, *Science and the Unborn* by Clifford Grobstein. Dr. Grobstein is by no means a man of evil intention. On the contrary, he is a biologist and embryologist of distinction who, we are assured by noted bioethicists, possesses exquisitely attuned ethical sensitivities. Grobstein knows that a great weakness of the pro-choice argument in the abortion debate is that it downplayed or dismissed concern about what it is, or who it is, that is being terminated in abortion. The American people, he recognizes, insist that that concern not be treated lightly. (A *New York Times*/CBS national poll published April 26, 1989, indicates that 16 years after the Supreme Court ruling, only 21% of those polled favor the policy of *Roe v. Wade.* Fully 48% think abortion is the same thing as murder. A *Boston Globe* poll a few weeks earlier had 57% identifying abortion as murder. We may well challenge the use of the term "murder," but do we really believe that ours would be a less violent, more caring and morally sensitive society if those people were less concerned about what or who is terminated in abortion?)

As a scientist, Grobstein acknowledges that even the zygote, and of course the embryo, is "human to the core." If abortion policy and policies that permit nontherapeutic experiments with the unborn are to be stabilized, they must be, he says, both rational and sensitive to the views of "a moral society." Religious beliefs opposed to what Grobstein proposes are deemed by him to be irrational, especially if they are Roman Catholic or fundamentalist (he tends to conflate the two). Therefore, a rational policy must finally be devised and implemented by experts in national and local commissions. Their task, says Grobstein, is one of "status assignment" with respect to who is and who is not to be treated as a person with rights. Not all who are given status assignment as human beings are also given "protective status assignment." It depends on how they come out when measured by an index of "quality of life." (*lebensunwertes Leben?*)

Those who are in charge of assigning status can also reassign status. Grobstein is primarily concerned about the treatment and uses of the unborn, but he acknowledges that his approach also has clear implications for the reassignment of the born, especially the elderly and gravely handicapped. Nonetheless, he assures us that "in the short term" the application of the approach he advocates can be limited to the early stages of life. It is important to note that the lethal use of the embryo, for example, does not diminish its human status, according to Grobstein. On the contrary, its human dignity is enhanced by its sacrifice of its life for the betterment of humanity through, for example, medical experiments and fertilization procedures.

A key component in Grobstein's argument deserves most particular attention. He acknowledges that even the "preembryo" has "biological membership in the human community" and must be respected for its "profound potential" to become "an individual in the fullest sense, an undeniable person." Such respect is appropriate "so long as [the unborn] has a reasonable probability of continuing development to become an infant and then an adult." But note: "The situation is transformed if, for whatever reason, a particular preembryo has no reasonable prospect of developing further." And why does it have no reasonable prospect of developing further? The answer is very simple: Because we have decided to terminate it. We have not deprived it of its potential life because, by virtue of our decision, it had no potential life. In that case, Grobstein writes, the unborn "need only be assessed and valued for its then-existing properties without reference to what it might have become in a normal human life history."

The doctrine being propounded could not be more clear: With respect to human dignity and human rights, the reality is what we define it to be. There are no prior rights that are there for us to respect. Rights are created by our assignment of rights. Grobstein explicitly states that the idea of "unalienable rights" endowed by Nature and Nature's God can have no place in bioethical discussions. As philosophers might put it, the objects of abortion, medical experimentation, and other measures have no ontological status. They may have a social-political status if we choose to assign them such status. They are what we agree to say they are. And the "we" who do the agreeing are, when it comes down to it, the experts who are capable of making rational definitions untainted by the religious and other prejudices of what Grobstein calls "the frozen past."

Why do I mention the book *Science and the Unborn*? Because it is recent and its author and argument are in the mainstream of current bioethical debates. We know they are in the mainstream because those who define the mainstream (e.g., Daniel Callahan and Richard McCormick) say they are in the mainstream. We might have chosen any number of other books or articles. It is not accurate to say that the argument advanced by Clifford Grobstein and others is reminiscent of the Nazi doctors. In critical respects, it is a replication of the argument advanced by the Nazi doctors. Those who remember, remember where they heard this kind of reasoning before. Dr. Karl Brandt and his colleagues argued this way almost 50 years ago. At Nuremberg, the civilized world rejected their argument. Now it seems that we are reconsidering that rejection. The suspicion may not be entirely unwarranted that, to the degree that we are reconsidering, we are the less civilized. Once again, I emphasize that the point here is not that abortion, embryo experiments, and other practices are morally equivalent to what was done in the Holocaust. There are many and important differences, and distinctions must be made. My point is simply that some justifying arguments for such practices today are very much like the arguments employed in the Holocaust, and that is reason for deepest concern.

In addressing "the use of metaphors and analogies concerning the Holocaust in contemporary bioethical debates," I have tried to limit myself to similar habits of mind and patterns of reasoning. There are many other analogies that might have been mentioned, each of them worthy of a paper in its own right. For instance, the euphemized vocabulary of death, by which we employ language that conceals from ourselves and others what we are doing and what we are proposing to do. For instance, the high stakes of wealth, power, and prestige that have been invested in current and developing technology and practice. And there is much else that is much like the Holocaust, but enough already.

I do not wish to end on a note suggesting despair. We should not grant Hitler a posthumous victory by succumbing to doctrines of historical or technological inevitability. Then is not now, there is not here, and they are not us. The banality of evil speaks of the everydayness of evil, of decisions made day by day, on days no doubt much like this day. And remembering the banality of evil can remind us also of the banality of virtue. Virtue, as Aristotle tells us, is a matter of habits, and, as Dr. Johnson tells us, a matter of remembering. Our time is not so new as we sometimes like to think. Demystified of the techniques and the professional jargon, the hard questions facing us today are, at their heart, the questions faced by the prophets of old. Who is my neighbor? To whom am I neighbor? Recognizing this truth does not give us the answer to all our bioethical debates, but it does keep before us the questions that we are answering.

The broken fences around the law can be repaired, and new fences can be erected. The safety rail surrounding the abyss can be strengthened. The signposts of Hippocrates and Nuremberg can be retrieved and refurbished. These things can be done; we cannot know whether they will be done. I confess that I draw encouragement from the way in which, in the last 16 years, a democratic people, opposing almost every establishment of the society, has refused to acquiesce in the lethal illogic of *Roe v. Wade*. But there is still a very long way to go. Every step we take is shadowed by the Holocaust. The way they were is, in important respects, ominously like the way we are. But that past need not be our future. The very holding of a conference on bioethics and the Holo-

caust may be taken as a sign of determination that that not
be our future. Never again? We simply do not know. We do
not need to know. Eliot had it right: "For us, there is only the
trying. The rest is not our business."

From: *When Medicine Went Mad* Ed.: A. Caplan
©1992 The Humana Press Inc.

The Abuse of Medicine
and the Legacy
of the Holocaust

Abuse of Human Beings for the Sake of Science

Jay Katz

Introduction

The third experiment...took such an extraordinary course that I called an SS physician of the camp as witness, since I had worked on these experiments all by myself. It was a continuous experiment without oxygen at a height of 12 kilometers conducted on a 37-year-old Jew in good general condition. Breathing continued up to 30 minutes. After 4 minutes the experimental subject began to perspire and wiggle his head, after 5 minutes cramps occurred, between 6 and 10 minutes breathing increased in speed and the experimental subject became unconscious; from 11 to 30 minutes breathing slowed down to three breaths per minute, finally stopping altogether.

Severest cyanosis developed in between and foam appeared at the mouth.

At 5 minute intervals electrocardiograms from three leads were written. After breathing had stopped Ekg (electrocardiogram) was continuously written until the action of the heart had come to a complete standstill. About 1/2 hour after breathing had stopped, dissection was started.[1]

Thus reads the report of Dr. Sigmund Rascher, a captain in the medical service of the German Air Force. He conducted this experiment in order to learn how long an aviator, falling through space without parachute and oxygen, would survive. "The experiments might result in death," he wrote in his initial proposal, and "nobody volunteers for them."[2]

The history of human experimentation testifies to medical science's extraordinary achievements to benefit humankind. Yet, that same history also bears witness to the abuse of human beings in the quest to advance knowledge. The concentration camp experiments highlight the most appalling and gruesome forms of abuse that can be inflicted on human beings, whenever the human rights of research subjects are utterly disregarded. When that happens, as the Rascher report illustrates, the immediate or soon-to-follow death of research subjects readily becomes a deliberate and integral part of the research design. This, to my knowledge, has never before or since been recorded in the annals of medical science.

Such abuse is unpardonable. Since it occurred, we must seek answers to many questions: Is any abuse of research subjects pardonable? What constitutes "abuse"? What kind of abuses are we willing to tolerate for the sake of scientific advancement?

If it is true that abuse of research subjects has stalked and still stalks the research enterprise, then it is wrong—dangerously wrong—to view the concentration camp experiments as solely the result of "the ravages of Nazi pseudo-science," as solely an isolated aberration in the history of medical experimentation. These experiments are an aberration in their unparalleled fiendish intensity, yet they are also an integral chapter in the history of thoughtless, ubiquitous, albeit milder and therefore, barely recognizable abuse of human beings for the sake of medical science.

As I wrote in the Introduction to *Experimentation with Human Beings*:

> When science takes man as its subject, tensions arise
> between two values basic to Western society: freedom

of scientific inquiry and protection of individual inviolability. Both are facets of man's quest to order his
world. Scientific research has given man some, albeit
incomplete, knowledge and tools to tame his environment, while commitment to individual worth and
autonomy, however wavering, has limited man's
intrusions on man. Yet when human beings become
the subject of experimentation, allegiance to one value
invites neglect of the other. At the heart of this conflict lies an age-old question: When may a society,
actively or by acquiescence, expose some of its members to harm in order to seek benefits for them, for
others, or for society as a whole?[3]

Harm here has two facets: harm to the integrity of the body
and harm to the integrity of personhood. I shall focus on harm
to the integrity of personhood; i.e., the harm inflicted by keeping human beings in the dark about any aspect of the research,
unless consented to by them. Underlying such practices is
the absence of an unwavering, uncompromising commitment by physician-scientists to placing disclosure and consent
above the claims of science. I shall argue throughout this chapter that without such a commitment, "voluntary consent"
is impossible; that without such a commitment, any definition of voluntary consent becomes compromised in application.

Human beings, I believe, can be invited to suffer harm
for the sake of advancing science, and their assent should
be honored. I equally believe that the vexing problem in
human research, from its beginnings to this date, has not
been exposure to physical harm. Instead, the problem has
been the infliction of harm to the integrity of personhood by
conscripting human beings into research without their consent;
by engineering consent through incomplete disclosure, double
talk, evasion, and fraud; by compelling consent through
exploitation of patient-subjects' necessitous circumstances.

In part two of this chapter I intend to place the concentration camp experiments in their historical and contemporary contexts. In part three, I identify the root causes that

made such experimentation inevitable and single out those
that have been endemic to the research enterprise. In part
four, I explore the question of whether the concentration camp
data should be relegated to oblivion or mined for their potential
to benefit humankind.

I am not trained to evaluate the significance of these
data for contemporary research. However, my reading of the
data makes me side with those who find valuable information in at least some of the experimental results. If the data
prove to be useless, the ethical dilemma of using the data
and thus benefitting from evil is moot, but not the questions
that the controversy over their use has raised: Can we benefit from evil without perpetuating evil? Can we disavow the
tree, if we are willing to grasp its fruit?[4] Are some deeds of
history so barbarous that to feast, by deliberate choice, on
their fruits makes cannibals of us all? Or is rejection of the
fruit, when humankind can benefit, a commensurate, or even
greater, evil?

The History of Human Experimentation

Experimentation Prior to 1933

The concentration camp studies had their antecedents.
Prior to 1933, published reports described French and German experiments in which cancerous tissue surgically removed
from one diseased breast was transplanted into the apparently healthy other breast; experiments with women, often
but not always prostitutes, whose healthy urethrae were
inoculated with gonococcus bacilli in order to prove that
"gonorrheic infection is one of the most important causes of
painful and serious afflictions of the sexual organs;" experiments with young men and women to demonstrate that the
secondary stage of syphilis is infectious; experiments with
newly born infants whose eyes were inoculated with tubercle
and gonorrhea bacilli in order to study the pathogenesis of
these organisms.[5]

Remarkable about these reports is not only that the experiments were carried out without consent or that they were performed on persons deemed inferior and powerless, but even more that the physician-scientists unselfconsciously confessed to their scientific cruelty and that no one who read their confessions protested. Consider:

> [The publication of these observations] will perhaps restrain others...from making further experiments, often leading to the complete wrecking of the lives of the persons subjected to them. It would add considerably to my peace of mind in respect to the victims' fate, if these experiments [were to establish the fact that the secondary stage of syphilis is contagious, so that] the sufferings of a few individuals were not too high a price to be paid by mankind for the attainment of such a truly beneficial and practical result.[6]

Or consider a Swedish investigator's justification for using young children as subjects for variola vaccine experiments:

> [P]erhaps I should have first experimented upon animals, but calves—most suitable for these purposes—were difficult to obtain because of their cost and their keep.[7]

The history of human experimentation, still to be written, will further document what all too briefly I have set forth here. Let me note only in passing that the treatment of research subjects, so often recruited from the patient population, has its antecedents in the treatment of patients. Indeed, it was this insight that led me from the study of human experimentation to the investigation of the physician-patient relationship. Myron Prinzmetal, while a medical student and resident in various American and European hospitals, recalled

> [the] degradation of a poor man with a prolapsed rectum who was asked to defecate in a wastebasket before the class in the proctology clinic...a poor young woman at the San Francisco County Hospital who was

stripped from the neck to knees in front of the entire class. Cringing with shame and embarrassment, she closed her eyes.[8]

Such egragious practices are now rare. Yet, they persist in more subtle, but equally humiliating, ways.

The Concentration Camp Experiments

I have already referred to the "high-altitude" or "low-pressure" experiments conducted at Dachau in 1942. I shall describe that and another experiment in somewhat greater detail to document what transpired in the concentration camps. Both were considered crucial to saving the lives of pilots and sailors.

The High-Altitude Experiments[9]

Early in the war it was deemed imperative to conduct research in the field of high altitude because of the higher ceilings reached by Allied fighter planes. The heights involved were 12,000–20,000 meters. Four series of experiments were first carried out: slow descent without oxygen, slow descent with oxygen, falling without oxygen, and falling with oxygen. The tests were designed to simulate either descent with parachute open or a free fall before the parachute opens. The experiments were also to determine whether the theoretically established norms of survival at high altitudes correspond with results obtained by practical experience.

Preliminary studies with parachute jumps had already demonstrated that lack of oxygen and low atmospheric pressure at 12 or 13 km altitude did not cause death. Fifteen experiments of this type had proven that whereas the subjects suffered from severe bends and unconsciousness, normal functions of the senses returned once they reached a height of 7 km on descent. Electrocardiograms, taken during these studies, registered temporary irregularities, but by the time the experiments were over the tracings returned to normal and remained so during subsequent follow-up studies.

However, obtaining data about the extent of bodily deterioration during repeated exposure to high altitude required a series of experiments that were lethal to the subjects. Such experiments were carried out and proved successful. They demonstrated that extreme deficiencies of oxygen can be endured. The secret report on these experiments, submitted by Dr. Sigmund Rascher on May 11, 1942, reads as follows:

> Based on results of experiments which up to now various scientists had conducted on animals only, the experiments in Dachau were to prove whether these results would maintain their validity on human beings.
>
> 1. The first experiments were to show whether the human being can gradually adapt himself to higher altitudes. Some 10 tests showed that a slower ascent without oxygen taking from 6 to 8 hours kept the functions of the senses of the various experimental subjects fully normal up to a height of 8,000 meters. Within 8 hours several subjects had reached a height of 9.5 kilometers without oxygen when bends occurred suddenly.
>
> 2. Normally it is impossible to stay without oxygen at altitudes higher than 6 kilometers. Experiments showed however that after ascent to 8,000 meters without oxygen, bends combined with unconsciousness lasted only about 25 minutes. After this period the subjects had mostly become accustomed to that altitude; consciousness returned, they could make knee bends, showed a normal electrocardiograph and were able to work (60 to 70 percent of the cases examined).
>
> 3. Descending tests on parachutes (suspended) without oxygen: These experiments proved that from 14 kilometers on down severest bends occurred which remained until the ground was reached. The detrimental effects caused by these experiments

manifested themselves at the beginning as unconsciousness, and subsequently as spastic and limp paralysis, catotomy, stereotypy, and as retrograde amnesia lasting several hours. About 1 hour after the end of the experiment the subjects for the most part were still disoriented as to time and locality. The blood picture often showed a shift to the left; albumen and red and white blood corpuscles were regularly found in the urine after the experiment; cylinders were sometimes found. After several hours or days, the blood and urine returned to normal. The changes of the electrocardiograph were reversible.

Contrary to descending tests on parachutes without oxygen, descending tests with oxygen were carried out from heights up to 18 kilometers. It was proved that on the average the subjects regained the normal function of their sense at 12 to 13 kilometers. No disturbances of general conditions occurred during any of these experiments. Brief unconsciousness at the beginning of the experiment caused no lasting disturbances. Urine and blood showed only a slight change.

4. As the long time of descent on parachutes, under actual conditions, would cause severe freezing even if no detrimental effects were caused by lack of oxygen, subjects were brought by sudden decreases in pressure with a cutting torch from 8 to 20 kilometers, simulating the damage to the pressure machine of the high altitude airplane. After a waiting period of 10 seconds, corresponding to stepping out of the machine, the subjects were made to fall from this height with oxygen to a height where breathing is possible. The subjects awoke between 10 and 12 kilometers and at about 8 kilometers pulled the parachute lever.

5. In experiments of falling from the same height without oxygen, the subjects regained normal function of their senses only between 2 and 5 kilometers.

6. Experiments testing the effect of pervitin on the organism during parachute jumps, proved that the severe after-effects, as mentioned under No. 3, were considerably milder. The ability to withstand the conditions at high altitudes was only slightly improved, while the bends, since they were not noticed, occurred suddenly (restraint-loosening effects of pervitin).

7. Dr. Kliches, of the Charles University in Prague, reports in the publication of the Reich Research Council: "By prolonged breathing of oxygen, human beings should theoretically be kept fully fit up to 13 kilometers. In practice, the limit is around 11 kilometers. Experiments which I carried out in this connection proved that with pure oxygen no lowering of the measurable raw energy (ergometer) was noticeable up to 13.3 kilometers. The subjects merely became unwilling since pains of the body cavities grew too severe, due to the lowering of pressure between body and thin air. When pure oxygen was inhaled bends occurred in all 25 cases only at heights above 14.2 kilometers."

As a practical result of the more than 200 experiments conducted at Dachau, the following can be assumed:

Flying in altitudes higher than 12 kilometers without pressure-cabin or pressure-suit is impossible even while breathing pure oxygen. If the airplane pressure-machine is damaged at altitudes of 13 kilometers and higher, the crew will not be able to bail out of the damaged plane themselves since at that height the bends appear rather suddenly. It must be requested that the crew should be removed automatically from the plane, for instance, by catapulting the seats by means of compressed air. Descending with opened parachute without oxygen would cause severe injuries due to the lack of oxygen, besides causing severe freezing; consciousness would not be regained until the ground was reached. Therefore the following is to be requested: 1.

A parachute with barometrically controlled opening.
2. A portable oxygen apparatus for the jump.

For the following experiments Jewish professional
criminals who had committed race pollution were used.
The question of the formation of embolism was investigated in 10 cases. Some of the subjects died during a
continued high-altitude experiment; for instance, after one half hour at a height of 12 kilometers. After
the skull had been opened under water an ample
amount of air embolism was found in the brain vessels and, in part, free air in the brain ventricles.

To find out whether the severe psychic and physical
effects, as mentioned under No. 3, are due to the formation of embolism, the following was done: After relative recuperation from such a parachute descending
test had taken place, however, before regaining consciousness, some subjects were kept under water
until they died. When the skull and the cavities of the
breast and of the abdomen had been opened under
water, an enormous amount of air embolism was found
in the vessels of the brain, the coronary vessels, and
the vessels of the liver and the intestines, etc.

That proves that air embolism, so far considered as
absolutely fatal, is not fatal at all, but that is reversible as shown by the return to normal conditions of all
the other subjects.

It was also proved by experiments that air embolism
occurs in practically all vessels even while pure oxygen is being inhaled. One subject was made to breathe
pure oxygen for 2 1/2 hours before the experiment
started. After 6 minutes at a height of 20 kilometers,
he died and at dissection also showed ample air
embolism, as was the case in all other experiments.

At sudden decreases in pressure and subsequent
immediate falls to heights where breathing is possible,
no deep reaching damages due to air embolism could
be noted. The formation of air embolism always needs
a certain amount of time.[10]

The Luftwaffe physicians appreciated that the experiments had left unconsidered the impact of excessive cold at
high altitude on the entire body. Since they believed that the
problems of both high altitude and freezing temperatures had
to be investigated separately, they subsequently conducted
experiments on the impact of freezing temperatures.

Prosecution witness Dr. Andrew C. Ivy, a distinguished
scientist at the University of Chicago Medical School, was
only partly correct when he testified at the Nuremberg trial
of the Nazi physicians that the desired information could have
been obtained from animals, for ultimate proof required
human experimentation. Yet his observations, in the context
of the Holocaust, were beside the point: Why not use human
beings first, when animals "were difficult to obtain because
of their cost and their keep."

The Sea-Water Experiments[11]

The sea-water experiments attempted to solve a question of importance to men of the Luftwaffe and Navy who
had to abandon their aircrafts or ships: Can sea water be
made potable and be ingested without detrimental impact to
health? One of the two known methods, the Schaefer method,
had been chemically tested and apparently produced potable
sea water. It had the disadvantage of requiring substantial
amounts of silver, which was in scarce supply. The second,
the so-called Berkatit method, employed a substance that
changed the taste of sea water but did not remove the salt. It
had the advantage of simplicity of manufacture and use.

However, preliminary studies had shown that "if the
Berkatit method is used, damage to health had to be expected
not later than 6 days after taking Berkatit [with resulting]

permanent injuries to health and [finally] death after not later than 12 days. [S]ymptoms [ranged from] dehydration, diarrhea, convulsions, hallucinations, and finally death."

To obtain more definitive data, new studies were conducted. They included a series of experiments, for a maximum of 6 or 12 days, during which one group was given sea water processed with Berkatit, another ordinary drinking water, another no drinking water at all, and a final group such water as was available in the emergency sea distress kits then used. It did not matter that the use of Berkatit caused permanent injuries to the research subjects by the sixth day and death no later than the twelfth day.

With respect to the studies' scientific merits, Dr. Franz Vollhardt, expert witness for the defense, contradicted, and correctly so, the assertion of Telford Taylor, Chief Prosecutor at the Nuremberg Trial, that "[t]hese experiments revealed nothing which civilized medicine can use."[12] Vollhardt, a distinguished German scientist asserted, "that scientifically speaking the planning was excellent." In response to a question of whether "these experiments [were] in the interests of aviators and sailors who [had been] shipwrecked," he stated that "towards the end of the war there was an increase in the number of pilots shot down as well as of shipwrecked personnel, and it was, therefore, the duty of the hygiene department...to consider the question of how one could best deal with cases of shipwrecked personnel..." He then added, "one unsuspected [finding of these studies turned out to be] that the drinking of small quantities of sea water, up to 500 cc over a lengthy period, [is] better than unalleviated thirst." Dr. Vollhardt finally expressed his conviction that the results of these experiments "were a wonderful thing for all seafaring nations."[13]

The lawyers for the defense repeatedly questioned Dr. Ivy on the ethical standards of human experimentation throughout the Western world. He correctly asserted that in American research—for example, on pellagra, yellow fever, beri-beri, and the plague—few deaths had occurred. Indeed, the two deaths reported in the yellow fever experiments involved physician-scientists who had experimented on themselves. Death as an explicit end-point of a research study, as I have emphasized, was never part of any methodology devised by other Western investigators.

However, Dr. Ivy evaded answering the question of whether other Western physician-scientists had committed moral indiscretions in the conduct of research. Instead of facing up to the existence of such indiscretions, he emphasized the impermissibility of such conduct:

> [The] moral responsibility that controls *or should control* the conduct of a physician should be inculcated into the minds of physicians just as moral responsibility of other sorts, and those principles are clearly depicted or enunciated in the oath of Hippocrates with which every physician *should* be acquainted.
>
> According to my knowledge, it represents the Golden Rule of the medical profession. It states how one doctor would like to be treated by another doctor in case he were ill. And in that way how a doctor *should* treat his patients or experimental subjects. He *should* treat them as though he were serving as a subject.
>
> Q: Several of the defendants have pointed out in this case that the oath of Hippocrates is obsolete today. Do you follow that opinion?
>
> A: I do not. The moral imperative of the oath of Hippocrates I believe is necessary for the survival of the scientific and technical philosophy of medicine.[14]

Note the repeated reference to "should." But the imperative of ethics does not necessarily reflect the reality of practice. Dr. Ivy perhaps knew that "should" is one thing and "do" another, for the ethical imperative advanced by him has been breached all too frequently in the practice of human

research. Moreover, as I shall soon contend, the Hippocratic
Oath is of little relevance to instructing physicians on how
to conduct themselves in the pursuit of the advancement of
medical science.

Experimentation in the US Since 1945

Any history of experimentation in the US prior to and
since the concentration camp experiments, whenever it is
written, will reveal more ubiquitous transgressions than
those that have come to our attention. Three of such studies
that have come to public awareness deserve brief comments.

The Beecher Expose[15]

In 1966, Henry K. Beecher, the renowned Dorr Professor of Research in Anesthesia at the Harvard Medical School,
discomforted the medical community by his assertion that
an "examination of 100 consecutive studies published in 1964
in an excellent journal [revealed that] 12 of these seemed to
be unethical." One of them reads as follows:

> The sulfonamides were for many years the only anti-
> bacterial drugs effective in shortening the duration of
> acute streptococcal pharyngitis and in reducing its
> suppurative complications. The investigators in this
> study undertook to determine if the occurrence of the
> serious nonsuppurative complications, rheumatic fever
> and acute glomerulonephritis, would be reduced by
> this treatment. This study was made despite the gen-
> eral experience that certain antibiotics, including peni-
> cillin, will prevent the development of rheumatic fever.
>
> The subjects were a large group of hospital patients; a
> control group of approximately the same size, also with
> exudative Group A streptococcus, was included. The
> latter group received only nonspecific therapy (no sul-
> fadiazine). The total group denied the effective peni-
> cillin comprised over 500 men.

Rheumatic fever was diagnosed in 5.4 percent of those treated with sulfadiazine. In the control group rheumatic fever developed in 4.2. percent.

In reference to this study a medical officer stated in writing that the subjects were not informed, did not consent and were not aware that they had been involved in an experiment, and yet admittedly 25 acquired rheumatic fever. According to this same medical officer more than 70 who had known definitive treatment withheld were on the wards with rheumatic fever when he was there.

The Jewish Chronic Disease Hospital Experiments[16]

In July 1963, three doctors, with approval from the director of medicine of the Jewish Chronic Disease Hospital in Brooklyn, New York, injected "live cancer cells" subcutaneously into 22 chronically ill and debilitated patients. The doctors did not inform the patients that they were participating in a research study designed to measure the patients' ability to reject foreign cells—a test entirely unrelated to their therapeutic program.

Eventually, the Attorney General of the State of New York charged the two doctors involved in the experiment with failure to obtain a valid and informed consent from the patients. Therefore, he alleged that the doctors were guilty of "fraud or deceit [and] the unprofessional practice of medicine." The Board of Regents of the University of the State of New York, which had jurisdiction over the imposition of sanctions for such transgressions, suspended the license of both physicians for one year, but stayed the execution of such suspensions on the condition that "they [now] conduct themselves in a manner befitting their professional status and [that they] conform fully to the moral and professional standards of conduct imposed by law and their profession..." The investigators' peers expressed their disdain about this most minimal sanction by electing the chief investigator of the study Vice President of the American Association for Cancer Research the year after sentence had been imposed, and its President the following year.

The problem with the Jewish Chronic Disease Hospital experiments was not so much that the injections of "live" cancer cells endangered the patients' physical well-being. That risk, if present at all, was minimal. Instead, the abuse was: that the patients were not told they were participating in an experiment completely unrelated to the treatment of the disease for which they had been hospitalized.

Many of the participants in the legal proceedings made light of this transgression. As one member of the subcommittee of the Committee on Grievances, which had been charged to consider the complaint, put it:

> The problems of informed consent are considered nebulous and insoluble by a large segment of competent medical authority. The emotional reaction to the word "cancer" very often justifies its concealment. The blind patient whose sight is restored is not informed that his or her new cornea was transplanted from a cancerous eye removed from another patient. There are other instances where significant facts are concealed from patients, concealment tolerated or condoned by both medical and civil authority.

Consider the conflation of treatment and research. Above all, consider the plea for concealment without any specification of its limits.

The Tuskegee Syphilis Study[17]

The Tuskegee Syphilis Study was conducted by physician-scientists of the US Public Health Service from 1932 to 1972. It was finally terminated on the recommendation of an Ad Hoc Advisory Panel, appointed in 1971 by Merlin DuVal, then Assistant Secretary of HEW. I was a member of this panel.

The story is frighteningly simple: Four hundred black males, suffering from syphilis, were deliberately left untreated for decades in order to study the natural history of untreated syphilis. The subjects were not informed of their participation in this project. Instead, they were led to believe that they were receiving special medical attention from Public Health Service physicians. Most, if not all, of the subjects, did not know that they had syphilis.

The duplicity perpetrated on the research subjects became even more egregious after the efficacy of penicillin in the treatment of syphilis had been established in the early 1940s. At that time, the Public Health Service investigators conspired with members of the local draft boards to have the subjects declared "4F," rather than their being inducted into the Armed Forces. Had they been drafted, Army doctors would have discovered the subjects' illness, treated their syphilitic condition, and, in turn, jeopardized the experiment.

The Ad Hoc Advisory Panel unanimously declared the study of untreated syphilis in male black subjects "ethically unjustified in 1932." It did so with reservations because the original 1932 protocols were at the time unavailable to us. I felt that a stronger indictment was warranted and wrote a concurring opinion, joined only by the late Dr. Vernal Cave:

> There is ample evidence in the records available to us that the consent to participation was not obtained from the Tuskegee Syphilis Study subjects, but that instead they were exploited, manipulated, and deceived. They were treated not as human subjects but as objects of research. The most fundamental reason for condemning the Tuskegee Study at its inception and throughout its continuation is...that [the subjects] were never fairly consulted about the research project, its consequences for them, and the alternatives available to them.

Our allegations were vindicated years later when the original research protocols had been unearthed. In our Concurring Opinion, we also noted that

[i]n theory if not in practice, it has long been, [as Claude Bernard wrote in 1865], "a principle of medical and surgical morality (never to perform) on man an experiment which might be harmful to him to any extent, even though the result might be highly advantageous to science," at least not without the knowledgeable consent of the subject. This was one basis on which the German physicians who had conducted medical experiments in concentration camps were tried by the Nuremberg Military Tribunal for crimes against humanity. Testimony at their trial by representatives of the American Medical Association clearly suggested that research like the Tuskegee Syphilis Study would have been considered intolerable in this country or anywhere in the civilized world. Yet, the Tuskegee study [began prior to the concentration camp experiments, was carried on during the Holocaust and] was not terminated after the Nuremberg findings and the Nuremberg Code had been widely disseminated to the medical community. Moreover, the study was not reviewed in 1966 when the Surgeon General of the USPHS promulgated his guidelines for the ethical conduct of research, even though this study was carried on within the purview of his department.[18]

Why such experiments? Any answers must encompass and account for the abuses perpetrated not only during the Nazi era but also prior and subsequent to the concentration camp research studies. Before attempting to provide answers, one issue that has obscured our vision needs to be identified: The crucial problem, as already noted, is not—although, of course, it can be a problem—that research subjects may suffer physical harm, or even death in the course of research.

Whereas the Nazi experiments caused harm and death and whereas American experiments—as demonstrated by the Beecher investigations and the Tuskegee Syphilis Study—jeopardized the quality of, or foreshortened the research subjects' lives, it must be remembered that these tragic outcomes in all these studies arose in settings of coercion, nondisclosure, and/or lack of concern for the fate of research subjects.

Today, the requirement of disclosure of risks can and does better control unconsented-to physical harm to subjects of research. However, the problem remains even with respect to physical harm; namely, that risk disclosures are understated because of a lack of thorough-going commitment to placing disclosure and consent above the claims of science. Such a lack of commitment affects conversation between physician-investigators and their patient-subjects in subtle but fateful ways. This problem will not be eliminated unless the problem of harm to the dignity of personhood is first addressed.

The Dantesque Inferno quality of the concentration camp experiments highlights what can happen when many of the treacherous roads to hell converge. On one of these roads human beings are subjected to harm to personhood, as evidenced in the Jewish Chronic Disease Hospital experiments where patients did not know that they served as subjects of research. In countless other experiments, physician-investigators, in their interactions with patient-subjects, have obfuscated the distinction between therapy and clinical investigation, have not been forthcoming about nonexperimental (therapeutic) alternatives to the proposed experimental treatment, or its randomness of assignment, its uncertainty of outcome. Such manipulations, however well-intended, in order not "to frighten" patient-subjects, constitute an abuse of person. They violate one aspect of the Hippocratic commandment "to abstain from whatever is deleterious and mischievous."[19]

Yet, the Hippocratic Oath has been correctly read to instruct physicians only "to follow that system of regimen, which according to my ability and judgment I consider for the benefit of my patients..."[20] Thus, at least for research, and for medical practice as well, a new oath must instruct physician-scientists that patient-subjects, to safeguard their personhood, should be consulted about the medical options available to them, that they cannot be allowed trustingly to submit to doctors' orders. Otherwise, physicians will continue to treat human beings as objects, stripping them of their personhood under the caring, yet ultimately destructive guise of safeguarding their "patienthood." Once that first step has been taken, respect for the person begins to be compromised. This problem will be addressed below.

The Concentration Camp Experiments and Human Experimentation in the Rest of the Western World— Comparative Perspectives

The Root Causes of the Concentration Camp Experiments

In this section, I attempt to identify the root causes of the concentration camp experiments and then, explore those that remain relevant to human research in a Naziless Western world. The following root causes account for the conduct of the Nazi physicians.[21]

Obedience to the Fuhrer who had ordered the extermination of Jews, Gypsies, and other "racially inferior" people. The solemn oath, taken by many Nazi physicians, read: "I swear to you, Adolf Hitler...loyalty and bravery. I pledge to you and to my superiors appointed by you, obedience unto death, so help me God."[22]

The ideology of race that proclaimed the superiority of the Aryan race, haunted by the fear that the biological, genetic purity of the Aryan race was imperilled by the admixture of foreign, tainted blood. This danger, the Nazis believed, could only be averted by the complete elimination of Jews, Gypsies, and ultimately all non-Nordic races. As Heinrich Himmler put it: The leadership's task is "like [that of a] plant-breeding specialist who, when he wants to breed a pure strain from a well-tried species that has been exhausted by too much cross-breeding, first goes over the field to cull the unwanted plants."[23]

Jews in particular were seen as agents of "racial pollution" and "racial tuberculosis."[24] Attitudes toward them were fuelled by a 2000-year history of antisemitism, and the fear that international Jewry was conspiring against the establishment of a 1000-year Reich. These religious and political concerns, reinforced by the Nazis' eugenic vision of "assembling and preserving the most valuable stocks of basic racial elements,"[25] made Jews triply unfit to remain part of the human race. The need for biological renewal, for purification of Aryan blood, required their extermination. Thus, the "Final Solution."

The ideology of science that was relentlessly committed to the idea of the advancement of knowledge for the benefit of mankind, now limited to the Aryan community. Consider that since the mid 19th century, the quest, the imperative to advance knowledge, had increasingly captivated the imagination of a small but influential group of physicians.

As described earlier, physicians then began to conscript indiscriminately patients as subjects for research. Yet, at the same time, they could not pursue their investigation with total disregard of the human beings involved. Now, during the Third Reich, a golden opportunity was presented to Nazi physician-scientists: to extend the frontiers of knowledge, to search for ultimate truths without constraint. Scientific questions of importance to unravelling the mysteries of life and illness could now be directly answered by using human beings as test animals. The ideology of science demanded that the opportunity be seized, since the human animals involved were worthless and would soon be exterminated anyway. Thus, why not use them to derive benefits for science and mankind? Imbued with the ethos of science, the scientific holocaust joined forces with the political holocaust.

The ethos of professionalism which asserted that patients' interests are best served by trusting their doctors and that trust means following doctors' orders. The Nazi physician-scientists brought to their endeavors their indoctrination in the ethos of Aesculapian authority.

Although during their medical education physicians had been taught the art of healing and even a caring concern for patients' physical well-being, they had also been taught that physicians must decide what is in their patients' best interests. They had not been educated to believe that patients be consulted, that patients' wishes be considered. Such revolutionary ideas were foreign to their thinking, as they had been—at least until most recently—to the thinking of physicians throughout the civilized world.[26]

Since curing was not seen as the joint responsibility of patient and physician but as a submission to the esoteric knowledge and, in turn, to the authority of the doctor, concentration camp inmates readily became patients who had to be protected from the ravages of "typhus epidemics" and fatal starvation. Thus, killing them was caring for them, performing *Therapia Magna Auschwitzciense* (T.M.A.). And T.M.A. readily shaded over to "doing things for science, learning things for [the sake of] science."[27]

The impact of the war on soldiers and civilians, which required finding solutions for the plight of drowning and thirsty sailors and airmen in icy seas, the plight of pilots forced to abandon their aircrafts at high altitudes, the plight of soldiers and civilians exposed to typhus and infected wounds inflicted by enemy bullets and bombs. Caring for them demanded finding answers to pressing medical questions of how best to treat them. Thus, the suffering and death of human beings served purposes of healing.

However unpardonable, the Nazi experiments attest to our inherent all-too-human capacities for aggression and evil, which have always compromised our capacities for love, caring, and goodness: and which can propel us to a descent into hell whenever our customary propensity to obey authority is represented by an authority that invokes "scientific" and "principled" reasons to reduce human beings to nonhuman status. Stanley Milgram warned us that his studies on *Obedience to Authority* revealed something more dangerous than anger, rage, and aggression; namely, "man's capacity to abandon his humanity, indeed, the inevitability that he does so, as he merges his unique personality into larger institutional structures."[28]

The confluence of these dynamic structures—Reich, party, medicine, science—made the concentration camp experiments inevitable. Fidelity to the Hippocratic Oath, Dr. Ivy's testimony notwithstanding, could not brake the onslaught of these powerful forces arrayed against it. Indeed, as has already been suggested, the Oath contributed to the dynamism of the concentration camp experiments by its emphasis on medical authority. Hippocrates declared that eradicating illness was the doctor's, and not the doctor's *and* the patient's responsibility. The doctor decides for the diseased patient and if the diseased patient is world Jewry, then the response by a Nazi physician to the question "how can you reconcile [killing] with your [Hippocratic] oath as a doctor" makes sense: "Of course I am a doctor and I want to preserve life. And out of respect for human life, I would remove a gangrenous appendix from a diseased body. The Jew is the gangrenous appendix in the body of mankind."[29] It can happen again. The next time it may be directed against other despised groups and for other root causes. If this were to happen, one can only hope that more physician-scientists— remembering the past and being educated differently from the way they have been previously—will resist.

The Root Causes
Still Operative in Human Research

To return to our world and to the question: Which of the root causes continue to exert an influence on the research enterprise and therefore contribute to any abuse of research subjects? I nominate two: the ideology of science and the ideology of the medical profession.

The Ideology of Science

J. Robert Oppenheimer vociferously and relentlessly opposed the development of the hydrogen bomb. Yet, when he testified before the US Atomic Energy Commission in 1954,

he made a startling admission during an exchange with the
Chairman of the Commission:

> Mr. Gray: Your deep concern about the use of the
> hydrogen bomb ... became greater, did it not, as the
> practicabilities became more clear? Is this an unfair
> statement?

> Dr. Oppenheimer: I think it is the opposite of true.
> Let us not say about use. But my feeling about devel-
> opment became quite different when the practicabili-
> ties became clear. When I saw how to do it, it was
> clear to me that one had at least to make the thing...[30]

Two basic characteristics, it has often been asserted,
underlie the origin and growth of science: "the need to control
the workings of nature for our welfare and the simple, irre-
ducible need to understand the world about us and ourselves."[31]

One need not quarrel with science's quest to advance
the frontiers of knowledge, even though fundamental questions about the ends of science still require careful thought,
as evidenced by the post World War II debate among atomic
scientists on the morality of their activities. However, my
focus is on the problem of scientific progress in situations
when human beings must be enlisted as research subjects.
In these instances, advancement of science should bow to a
greater principle: protection of individual inviolability. The
rights of individuals to thorough-going self determination and
autonomy should come first. Scientific advances may be
impeded, perhaps even become impossible at times, but it is
a price worth paying.

Implementation of such a principled position would
require a massive shift in the attitudes of medical scientists.
To be sure, they are more sensitive than they have ever been
to the rights of research subjects. However, what they now
have learned is to "balance" the prerogatives of research subjects against the importance of the research project, the physical risks involved, and so forth. But in this balancing of the
ethic of science to advance knowledge against the ethic of

beneficence to benefit mankind, the latter ethic continues to loom large in their minds. Thus, any concern over the impact of research on research subjects becomes readily infiltrated by the claims of the ideology of science. We must cease to balance.

Instead, I propose a different scenario: A first and thorough-going commitment to unequivocal honesty in making disclosures to the subjects of research, a willingness to abandon a contemplated research project if too many subjects do not volunteer after all alternatives, risks, and benefits have been explored with them.

This suggestion should not be viewed as another definition of informed consent. Such a new definition is premature. It will be easier to formulate once, and if, this proposal is accepted. For now, I only want to give some concrete content to what respect for persons dictates if it were to become the polestar of interactions between physician-scientists and their research subjects.

Only once such a commitment has become deeply ingrained in physician-scientists' individual and collective psyche and they, in turn, view the advancement of science as a secondary objective, will they be able to stop talking about how "to comply" with informed consent requirements. Only then will they cease to treat such requirements as onerous obligations. Only then will the immediate preoccupation with research methodology, as soon as the research question has been formulated, yield to a preoccupation with prior questions: Can the contemplated project be presented honestly to patient-subjects? Can such a presentation be made with fidelity to respect for person? Thus, a change in research-scientists' basic belief system is required that says not: think advancement of science first, but think fidelity to human beings first.

To be more specific, the elders of the medical profession, who now instruct the next generation of physician-scientists, must set an example, by word and deed, that human beings come first. Medical schools must neither base faculty salaries on abilities to generate research grants, nor base promotion on the quantity of scientific papers; for some projects will have to be abandoned, once the existing pressure to conscript human subjects into research participation is eliminated. It may then take more time to enlist the requisite number of subjects and the rate of publications may suffer. As one research-physician recently told a class of medical students, in an attempt to justify tampering with informed consent requirements, "I have to get research grants to pay my and my laboratory assistants' salaries. I have to get results in order to generate new grant money and to secure my advancement."

I propose this in the shadow of the concentration camp experiments, but not to suggest that any departure from my prescription or even the continuation of existing practices turn scientist-physicians into Nazis. To think that would constitute an egregious and offensive misunderstanding of my position. To become Nazi scientists requires the confluence of forces that do not exist in our society.

What is conveyed here is more subtle and more troubling because of its subtlety: that the ideology of science, if given primacy, inexorably leads to disregard of respect for personhood. It is difficult to distinguish between ends and means unless one is clear about the ends first. Only then can the means be specified. The traditional ends of science in research with human beings need to give way to a new end: respect for the person.

Whereas such a fundamental reorientation will create formidable problems, it will not destroy the research enterprise. Instead, it will compel finding new and creative alternatives to customary research practices. Research subjects will continue to participate in research but they will do so now in a true collaborative spirit. Whether this prediction will turn out to be wrong, only time can tell. Scientists have had too little experience with interacting with research subjects in the spirit of these recommendations.

A Bridging Comment

Before turning to the ideology of the profession, an encounter far removed from the investigator-subject relationship, will illuminate my insistence on giving preeminence to respect for person. Janet Malcolm's article "The Journalist and the Murderer"[32] provides a useful text for highlighting the problems identified in the previous and next sections.

The facts are these: After his arrest for the murder of his wife and children, Dr. Jeffrey MacDonald and his attorney agreed to let Joe McGinniss participate in trial preparation. After his conviction, MacDonald—having good reasons to believe that McGinniss believed in his innocence—agreed to a series of candid interviews and an exchange of correspondence with McGinniss. McGinniss then wrote a book, *Fatal Vision*, which also found MacDonald guilty of murder. MacDonald sued McGinniss for "soul murder." At the trial, MacDonald attempted to prove that in inviting and assisting McGinniss in writing a book about him, he had every expectation that McGinniss would defend his innocence; and that McGinniss had shamelessly deceived him throughout, and subsequent to, the trial, by making him believe that McGinniss did not doubt his innocence. Many of McGinniss' letters to MacDonald supported that contention. During the trial, the tension between McGinniss' deception, on the one hand, and a journalist-writer's freedom of speech, on the other, were hotly contested. A number of journalists testified on behalf of McGinniss, including William F. Buckley, Jr. and Joseph Wambaugh.

Here are excerpts from McGinniss' testimony. In response to the question, "you didn't feel that you in any sense betrayed Jeffrey or did him dirt?," he sidestepped the question by answering: "My only obligation from the beginning was to the truth." On cross-examination, McGinniss reiterated his basic position: "I believe because I was encouraging him to not discourage me from finishing the book that I had put so much of my life into at that point. My commitment was to the book and to this truth."

Joseph Wambaugh agreed:

In writing, "The Onion Field," I can recall one of the murderers asking me if I believed him when he said he didn't shoot the policeman, and I at that time had interviewed scores of witnesses and had a mountain

of information, and I did not believe him, but I said
that I did, because I wanted him to continue talking.
Because my ultimate responsibility was not to that
person, my responsibility was to the book.

MacDonald's lawyer, in his closing statement, observed:

What's outrageous is that the defendant here, supposedly the protector of the First Amendment free-
doms—freedom of speech, freedom of expression—has
put experts on the stand who said, in Mr. Kornstein's
own words, that they must do whatever is necessary
to write the book. Those were the words that he used:
"whatever is necessary."

Those words have been used by dictators, tyrants,
demagogues throughout history to rationalize what
they have done. We've just gone through a series of
Congressional investigations where that was also one
of the excuses: We had to do what was necessary. It
was alright to lie, because it was necessary.

Janet Malcolm concluded her article with these observations:

Unlike other relationships, which have a purpose
beyond themselves and are clearly delineated as such
(dentist-patient, lawyer-client, teacher-student), the
writer-subject relationship seems to depend for its life
on a kind of fuzziness and murkiness, if not utter
covertness, of purpose. If everybody put his cards on
the table, the game would be over. The journalist must
do his work in a kind of deliberately induced state of
moral anarchy.

Malcolm's account illustrates the conflicting tensions
between a commitment to the person, on the one hand, and
the truth, the book, on the other, as well as the inevitable
consequences whenever the conflict remains unresolved. It
also highlights the human proclivities to deception of self and
others in the quest for personal success and/or respect for
one's craft. McGinniss and his journalist-witnesses argued

that deception was required and professionally justified. Even if correct, what McGinniss did constituted an abuse of person.

In human research, similar tensions exist between a commitment to respect for the person vs the "pursuit" of scientific truths in the service of advancing knowledge. Any balancing of these tensions compels, as it did in McGinniss' case, if not deliberate deception, then unconscious evasion, falsification, and omission of pertinent information. It cannot be otherwise. That is the reason why such practices will not cease unless respect for person becomes the guiding principle.

What transpires now in interactions between physician-scientists and patient-subjects may not rise to "moral anarchy," but it does rise to moral confusion. In passing, I would like to note one disagreement with Malcolm's views. She writes that "[t]he journalist, [unlike the dentist, lawyer, teacher (she does not mention physicians)] must do his work in a kind of deliberately induced state of anarchy." To the contrary, what she calls "moral anarchy" extends to the conduct of all professions, including physician-scientists.

The Ideology of the Medical Profession

The 30-year-long debate on greater patient participation in decision making, stimulated by law's promulgation of the informed consent doctrine in 1957, should not obscure the fact that throughout medical history, physicians have believed that patients' welfare is best protected if they follow doctors' orders. The concept of patient autonomy, until recently, was not part of the vocabulary of medicine. Whereas in today's world patients are provided with more information than they have been in the past, many of the real obstacles to patients' fuller participation in decision making have neither been addressed, nor, of course, overcome. The preface to the paperback edition of my book *The Silent World of Doctor and Patient* addresses these issues.

> My critics' second contention that significant improvements have occurred in the physician-patient dialogue dismisses too lightly the central arguments of my book: (1) that meaningful collaboration between physicians and

patients cannot become a reality until physicians have
learned how to treat their patients not as children but
as the adults they are; how to distinguish between
their ideas of the best treatment and their patients'
ideas of what is best; and how to acknowledge to their
patients (and often to themselves as well) their ignorance and uncertainties about diagnosis, treatment,
and prognosis; and (2) that medical educators have
failed to prepare future physicians for the responsi-
bilities that shared decision making imposes... Medical educators need to appreciate more than they do
that learning how to converse with patients is as difficult a task as learning about diseases, their patho-
physiology, diagnosis, and treatment. As Franz Kafka
observed, "[t]o prescribe pills is easy but to reach an
understanding with people is very hard."[33]

It will take time, if the time ever comes, for patients to
assume a more central role in deciding their medical fate. A
2000-year tradition is difficult to reverse and requires a
major shift in the ideology of professionalism. There may be
occasions when paternalism has a place in the practice of
medicine, but invocation of the principle of beneficence, which
informs resort to paternalism, must at least withstand a prior
relentless scrutiny of the primary principle: patient self-
determination. As long as patients are viewed as significantly
impaired to make decisions on their own behalf, the danger
is great that patient-subjects' autonomy in research decision
making—particularly in clinical research—will remain
equally threatened.

To summarize: Two of the root causes that affected the
conduct of the Nazi physician-scientists have similarly affected
human research throughout its history. If the balancing of
respect for persons against the ideologies of science and
professionalism continues, it should at least be recognized
what such a balancing entails: at least some inroads on
respect for personhood.

Benefiting from Evil

Should the data obtained from the Nazi concentration camp experiments be exploited for our benefit? I shall address this question in two ways: (1) How I would answer it if I were a scientist, confronted with such a decision, and (2) what professional and societal restrictions, if any, should be imposed on the use of the data?[2]

To begin with personal history, last year I was invited to write an op-ed article on this question. The invitation followed widely circulated newspaper reports on a decision by Lee Thomas, head of the US Environmental Protection Agency, to bar the use of any data acquired from experimentation on concentration camp inmates.[34] The data came from lethal experiments with phosgene gas that were designed to find an antidote to this highly poisonous substance.

Phosgene gas was widely employed as a chemical weapon during World War I. It causes irritation of, and fluid accumulation in the lungs, making breathing difficult, if not impossible. Today, phosgene is widely used in the manufacturing processes of plastics and pesticides. About one billion pounds are produced annually in the US. Thus, the EPA is concerned about the health risks to which both plant workers and people living near factories are exposed. I.C.F. Clement Inc., an environmental consulting firm, utilized the Nazi data while undertaking a risk assessment of the chemical for EPA. After 22 EPA employees had signed a letter of protest, Lee Thomas barred their use.

The critics asserted that "to use such data debases us all as a society, gives such experiments legitimacy, and implicitly encourages others...to perform unethical experiments." They also claimed that the experiments were so poorly designed that the data were worthless. A number of people at EPA and the consulting firm strongly disagreed. One of them stated, "of course, nobody in their right mind condones the experiments. The question is, given that this fiendish thing was done, what do you do with the information that exists? I suspect that the concentration camp inmates would have wanted to have the information used to help somebody."[35]

The Nazi data are the only available experimental information on the effect of phosgene on human beings. Although the experiments allegedly were poorly designed, the data are considered to be useful. An EPA toxicologist insisted that similar information, coming, for example, from an industrial accident exposing workers to the chemical, would prove invaluable. He then went on to say, "my personal opinion is that when data is collected in an unethical fashion, if it is important in protecting public health and is not available in any other way, I would use it."

One of my critics, in response to the op-ed article I eventually wrote, asked: "Is it fair to those people currently being exposed to the chemical to pretend that applicable data do not exist? Can the ethical questions be so compelling that we ignore information that might conceivably reduce the amount of human suffering and misery currently being experienced?"

Note one of the contradictory points already made: The experiments are useless, the experiments are invaluable. I have studied these experiments and, as I have already suggested, I believe that they contain valuable information. If not, there is no problem to be considered. Also note the question: "Can the ethical questions be so compelling to ignore this information?" I have thought about this question. My answer is: "Yes, ethical considerations can be that compelling."

When I first received the invitation to write the op-ed article, I thought that I would answer the question affirmatively, i.e., that I would defend the use of the data. In my prior work, I had always taken the position—contrary to many others, including editors of scientific medical journals— that unethically obtained data should be published, not so much for reasons of their scientific contributions to the cure of disease but for two different reasons: (1) to alert the scientific community and the public to the fact that unethical research is still being conducted. Without such an awareness, unethical practices will not come under better control; and

(2) to bring the offending medical scientists before duly authorized committees that will review their conduct and impose sanctions, severe ones, if indicated. Of course, I was often praised for my views on publication and criticized for my views on sanctions. I soon realized that my reasons for publishing contemporary unethically conducted research had no relevance to the question before me because the Nazi experiments (1) are part of history and no one questions that they were unethical and (2) the physicians involved have been held accountable and punished.

After agonizing over the question posed—writing draft after draft and being mindful of having to express my views in 750 words—I finally concluded that the data should not be used.

The article was widely reprinted. The published version departed, for a variety of reasons, from the original one. Excepts from the original draft read as follows:

> The conduct of the Nazi physician-scientists was barbarous, revolting, monstrous, devoid of any decency. Their research defiled human beings, medicine, science and humanity. They dragged through bloody mud an honorable profession to which contemporary physician-scientists who now wish to make use of these results belong.
>
> My answer is this: Whatever the benefit to mankind, the results of the experiments should be condemned to oblivion. The experiments' only benefit resides in bringing them, with results omitted, to the attention of the world ...
>
> Before giving my reasons, let me state what my reasons are not: I do not believe that in using the results we condone the experiments; whatever we do with the data, the experiments cannot be condoned. Nor do I believe that by publishing the results, we invite their repetition; for if ever repeated, the world will have descended into hell once again, and then nothing will save us. Nor do I believe that using the data with

appropriate acknowledgement of their source, can truly etch onto our minds the horrors of what had transpired; for deriving benefits from them will compel us immediately to suppress their origins, out of guilt over having benefited from such bloody deeds. Nor do I believe that we give a shred of meaning to the victims' lives and suffering by using the data; for we are dishonoring them even more by feasting on their bodies.

These experiments should never have been conducted. These results should never have been obtained. Let us not forget that.

Thus, my reason for not using the data for our benefit is this: Their use may dehumanize us as conducting the experiments did the Nazi physicians.

The reactions to the article were varied, often very intense. While teaching a course on Professional Responsibility at Yale Medical School, I read my statement to the medical students. The class was divided in its response: great praise, severe criticism. I noted a gender difference: Many of the female medical students liked what I had said, many of the male medical students were most critical.

I received many letters, one of which argued: "to follow your logic, we should not benefit from many architectural monuments—like the pyramids—because they were built with slave labor under the most inhumane conditions."

It was hard to write what I did in 750 words. But now I can expand on what I said then.

On reflection, mine was a most personal reaction, influenced by what the Nazis had done to my relatives, to my people. I now ask myself: Would I have reacted similarly if the data had come from Armenian, Chinese, Pakistani research subjects, or if the experiments had been conducted a century earlier? I continue to ask myself this question because I know how easy it is to become insensitive to the suffering of those to whom we are not intimately related. Freud spoke of the "narcissism of minor differences"[36] that reinforces human beings' inclination to aggression. And if not to aggression, then at least to indifference. Between strangers, *homo homini lupus* (man is a wolf to man).

Although I would not make use of the data, what about others? Consider first that the concentration camp research data are in the public domain. They are available to anyone. Thus, to prohibit their use requires state action. In arguing against their use, I do not wish to endorse governmental censorship. I am opposed to state censorship.

At the same time, a different form of "censorship" or disapproval would not concern me: the refusal of editors of scientific journals to publish articles that made use of such data or statements by scientific organizations advising their colleagues that the data should not be used.

At a minimum, journal editors and scientific organizations should insist that any article that made use of the data include a sufficiently detailed description of where they came from, including their blood- and tear-soaked history. They should also insist that the author set forth why he resolved the ethical dilemma in favor of using the Nazi data. Merely referring by a footnote, as has often been done, to the "Dachau experiments," is not enough.

Ultimately, the individual conscience of investigators must decide whether to use the data or not. However, investigators need to remain aware that in making use of the data, they force science to confront an examination of its own values. Science is not value-free, as the tension between advancement of science and protection of the inviolability of the subjects of research demonstrates. The often advanced claim that science is totally objective, and that therefore, the Nazi data "are merely objective scientific findings," constitutes a cruel deception of self, science, and the subjects of research. It denies that the data are soaked in blood, agony, and death.

Thus, in using the data, scientists make a political, as well as a scientific, decision. There is a distinction between developing a hydrogen bomb and using it. When Oppenheimer testified before the US Atomic Energy Commission, after admitting—as already quoted—that one "had to at least make [the hydrogen bomb]," he went on to say, "[t]hen the only problem was what would we do about them when one had them."[37] We have the Nazi experimental data. The question is now before us: What shall we do with them? This is not only, if it is at all, a scientific judgment; it is foremost a political one.

However hard one may try, one cannot separate the data from the way they were obtained. If science eschews the Nazis' scientific methodology of subject selection and treatment, the question must be faced: Should a judgment of unacceptable methodology relegate the findings to oblivion as they would be if the judgment were made that the research was so faulty that the results were worthless?

One dangerous proposition, advanced by some commentators and scientists in an attempt to isolate the Nazi from all other research studies, can be put to rest: That "experiments which are ethically unsound are also scientifically unsound." If that proposition were true, then many experimental studies conducted throughout the world would be unsound and invalid. This is just not so.

My reasons, my own personal history notwithstanding, for not using the data are difficult to put into words. Perhaps a quote from an article that I wrote when asked to speak on my role in the history of the regulation of human research will shed some light on why I feel the way I do.

> As I reflect about the history of human experimentation, I find in it much that attests to the perseverance, idealism, and sacrifice of investigators. We can only admire and be grateful to these intrepid pioneers. At the same time, I also can find in this history much that is sordid, frightening, and unconscionable. That this is so should come as no surprise. The abuses only testify to the all-too-human proclivities for aggression. Physicians and researchers are not exempt from these dynamisms. Indeed, they are particularly vulnerable

to them because their dedication to the advancement of science can blind them to the human costs of research. Denials and rationalizations are powerful allies of aggression.

If we wish to honor the victims of Auschwitz, we must appreciate that the cruel experiments conducted there cannot be attributed solely to the ravages of Nazi pseudo-science or to the Nazi physicians themselves. Auschwitz only revealed, and more starkly than ever, the capacity for aggression inherent in all of us.[38]

Yet, we must also remind ourselves that in the history of human experimentation, nothing compares with the deeds of the Nazi physicians. It is this difference that makes the Auschwitz and Dachau experiments so cruelly unique.

In the literature on medical practice, the problem of physicians maintaining their empathic identifications with patients, on the one hand, and a sense of detachment, on the other, has received considerable attention. All too often, detachment—however understandably, however sadly—overwhelms empathic concern. In using the data, scientists must consider the violence they could do to their empathic feelings. If this might be true, they should at least recognize that danger and not hide behind "the scientific objectivity" of their intentions. If they at least did that, they might be able to contain the tragic choices they are making in this instance and prevent their spilling over into other areas of their work.

We have not been very successful in containing human aggression and evil. Perhaps this is an instance when we can do so by proclaiming and at a personal price—to mankind and personal advancement—that we shall not use the data, that we shall suffer too, as the victims did.

Thus, the real and nagging questions are: Can we simultaneously repudiate and benefit from evil? In choosing to benefit from evil and making it part of our own history, will we perpetuate evil? As Edmond Cahn once put it, "[t]o possess the end and yet not be responsible for the means, to grasp the fruit while disavowing the tree, [that has throughout the ages been mankind's] chief hypocrisy."[39]

In re-immersing myself in the account of the concentration camp experiments, I experienced considerable pain as a person who lost many relatives in the Holocaust, and great anguish, as a physician, in arguing that the experimental data should not be used for the benefit of humankind. Now, two and one-half years have passed since I presented this chapter as a paper at the University of Minnesota. In the meantime I have changed my mind on the use of the data, and I intend to present my reasons in a forthcoming book on historical and contemporary aspects of human experimentation. In this chapter I decided not to modify the arguments I made then because I believe they have merit, my change of mind notwithstanding. There are no final answers to these tragic questions. I do not know whether five years hence I may not embrace once again what I have set forth here.

From: *When Medicine Went Mad* Ed.: A. Caplan
©1992 The Humana Press Inc.

"Medspeak" for Murder

The Nazi Experience and the Culture of Medicine

William E. Seidelman

Nazi medicine challenges the ethical foundation of medicine today. Whereas the genesis of bioethics occurred in the ashes of Nazi Germany, modern medicine has been unable or unwilling to recognize the enormity of the role played by medicine in Nazi Germany, or the implications of that role for medicine and medical science today. Nazi medicine was neither an aberration that arose in 1933 and disappeared in 1945, nor was it an anomaly relevant only to Nazi Germany and German-occupied Europe. Nazi medicine had its origins in the same academic and professional environment that influenced the development of the health care systems of the developed world. It was created and developed in the birthplace of scientific medicine: 19th and 20th Century Germany. The German medical school, which served as a model for medical education in North America, is the same medical school that graduated physicians who became practitioners of evil. Nazi medicine thrived in the health care system that gave the world socialized medicine. It did not die on the gallows at Nuremberg; its influence continues to this very day.

Nazi medicine eroded the foundation of medical practice, the relationship of the physician to human life. Medicine could achieve a better understanding of that relationship by studying its pathology through a dissection and analysis of the worst hour in the history of the profession: 1933–1945. The pathological sequelae of Nazi medicine can be described through an examination of its impact on the culture of medicine; a culture based on language, symbols, specialized institutions, and a unique form of social hierarchy.

Language

Medical culture has its own formal vocabulary that defines organ systems and diseases. It also has its own informal colloquial language and euphemisms or "medspeak" that is incorporated into the language of this conference such as "medicalized killing," "euthanasia," "medical experiments." In the context of Nazi medicine, these three terms are "medspeak" for murder. "Medicalized killing" in Nazi Germany was state-inspired murder. The genocidal process of Nazi Germany probably would not have achieved what it did without the legitimization and active complicity of the medical profession. Through the program of medical murder, physicians defined, selected, experimented on, and killed the victims. Physicians designed the instruments of death and exploited the victims' bodies before, during, and after their murders.[1–3] This program of mass murder began when physicians decided that human life was of differential value; when race became a metaphor for disease. The penultimate expression of the medicalization of human destruction is exemplified by the "medspeak" of Auschwitz, where physicians described the gas chamber/crematorium as the "Great Hospital" where the "patients" received the "Great Therapy of Auschwitz," death in the gas chamber.[4] The metaphorical Jew as disease received his metaphorical cure in the extermination center.

An important part of the medical process of rationalizing murder was the concept of human degeneration that defined some human beings as clinically degenerate "useless eaters" or "life without value."[5] In Nazi Germany, these concepts became legitimate expressions of clinical judgment. Murder was rationalized on the basis of clinical dehumanization.

Although the language of medicine today may exclude the concept of medical murder, the vernacular "medspeak" of the wards of our teaching institutions includes words synonymous with the concept of degeneration. The colloquial "medspeak" of students and housestaff in our health sciences centers today includes such expressions as "GOMER" and "SHPOS," expressions that imply some human beings are of lesser value than others.[6,7]

Thus, the language of medicine today exemplifies a dichotomy: an implicit acceptance of degeneracy and a denial of the concept of medical murder. By tolerating the "medspeak" of degeneracy and yet denying the reality of medical murder in Nazi Germany, the medical profession of today is exhibiting a naivete that threatens to further undermine the ethical basis of medical practice. Physicians must recognize the professional potential for evil, its antecedents and its endpoint. By ignoring the continued existence of the former and denying the latter, the culture of medicine today exhibits behaviors that suggest the profession has yet to achieve the maturity and wisdom necessary to establish an impermeable ethical foundation that will preserve the sanctity of the relationship of the physician to human life. The language of medical culture must consider the reality of its history and the value of that relationship.

Symbols

The culture of medicine has many symbols. They include a bust of Hippocrates, the staff of Aescelapius, and portraits of luminaries from the distant and recent past such as Galen, Vesalius, Lister, and Osler. A symbol of modern medicine is a physician's license to practice, usually found hanging on the wall of the physician's office. In most countries, the medical license represents state and professional approval of a graduate physician's qualifications. It symbolizes trust in the physician for the patients who attend such a person. That symbol was shattered on the selection ramp at Auschwitz. Benno Müller-Hill has pointed out that the SS physicians who selected people on the ramp in the Birkenau death camp were required to be licensed practitioners.[8] Thus, the medical license as a symbol of respect and trust became a symbol of death and destruction. In Nazi Germany it became a qualification for murder.

During the Hitler period, medical licensure took on a broader perverse meaning. It became a method of professional control and discrimination within and outside Germany. Within Germany, those physicians defined as racially inferior were deprived of their license to practice medicine. Outside Germany, many countries used the licensing process to deprive refugee physicians from the most scientifically advanced country in the world from the opportunity to practice their profession. In prewar France, the US, Australia, and the British Mandate of Palestine, the medical license became a symbol of discrimination and control.[9-17] Recently in West Germany, control of licensure was used as a form of professional suppression. In that country, a physician in Mainz had his license to practice suspended for having published a 1986 English language article in *Lancet* which raised ethical questions concerning the German medical professions' role in Nazi Germany.[18,19]

Thus, a modern symbol of medical culture, the medical license, has also come to represent a dichotomy: trust and evil. The Nazi period demonstrated the vulnerability of medical practice to state control by virtue of the license to practice. The license became a vehicle for, and thus a symbol of, professional and state controlled discrimination. That symbol of medical culture was used, not to promote the well-being of the individual patient, but to facilitate the malevolent goals of the state and the profession.

Institutions

In the culture of scientific medicine, the institution of the medical school symbolizes excellence; the best of education, medical science, and medical practice. It was to the German university-based medical schools that physicians made pilgrimages in pursuit of scientific and clinical excellence. It was the German university that the American educator, Abraham Flexner, saw as a model for his visionary health-science centers.[20] Many of these German universities saw their faculty receive Nobel prizes for contributions to medicine. It was also these same medical schools that employed the professors who legitimized Nazi racial policies and rapidly incorporated racial science into their curriculum.[21] The physicians Joseph Mengele and Sigmund Rascher, as well as the other licensed SS physicians who took their turn on the ramp at Auschwitz, were graduates of the German university.

The dichotomy of German medicine, scientific progress and evil, is exemplified by the recent discovery of the continuous use of the remains of Nazi victims as anatomical specimens by at least three German universities: Tübingen, Heidelberg, and Cologne. In addition, two German research institutions, the Max Planck Institute for Brain Research and the Vogt Collection, have been found to contain brain specimens derived from victims of the Nazi's euthanasia program.[22-25] The utility of science appears to have taken precedence over human decency. Thus, the German university as a symbol of excellence has been tainted by both its promotion of racism during the Hitler period and its continuous exploitation of evil, over four decades after the defeat of the Hitler regime and the Nuremberg War Crimes Tribunal.

We cannot dismiss those German institutions and their values as being irrelevant to us. They are part of our own heritage. The questions we ask of them concerning their basic value system we should also be asking of ourselves. We acknowledge the nobility of this heritage but we ignore the ignobility. The anatomical specimens in these German institutions symbolize the ignobility of medicine. The establishment of an ethical foundation in medicine requires that the profession recognize and acknowledge evil and pay tribute to its victims. We should begin in the symbolic birthplace of modern scientific medicine: the German university.

The Academic Hierarchy

The culture of the profession is defined by the academic hierarchy. In Nazi Germany, it was the leaders of the academic hierarchy, the professors, who provided the scholarly justification for medical murder and took advantage of the program of dehumanization and medicalized murder to advance their own personal scientific careers. It was these same professors who established the role models for young physicians in pursuit of academic careers.

Two professors who scaled the heights of academic distinction in the German university, Ernst Rüdin and Otmar von Verschuer, exemplify the sardonic nature of the culture of the academic hierarchy of Nazi medicine and its continuing influence.

Ernst Rüdin—Psychiatry and Human Genetics

Ernst Rüdin was a leading psychiatric geneticist whose particular field of interest was the genetics of schizophrenia. In 1916, he was the author of a paper that suggested schizophrenia was hereditary.[26] Rüdin subsequently became a professor of psychiatry at the University of Munich and director of the Kaiser-Wilhelm Institute of Psychiatry in Munich. Rüdin's research into the genetics of schizophrenia served as a foundation for his leadership in developing the eugenic and racist policies of the Hitler regime. He was one of the authors and advocates of the 1933 sterilization law. Rüdin viewed the Nuremberg race laws as being a victory for his eugenics movement. At Rüdin's Munich institute, to be a conscientious-objector was considered a form of schizophrenia and therefore a qualification for enforced sterilization.[27,28]

Today, Rüdin's early work on the genetics of schizophrenia continues to be cited without any consideration of the context of this work or the career of the medical scientist responsible. An example of this occurred recently in *Nature*, which published four papers dealing with the genetics of schizophrenia. Rüdin's 1916 paper was cited in one of these papers without any consideration of the historical context of his work.[29,30] Ernst Rüdin's work and career exemplify the achievement of an academic physician and scientist who achieved distinction in a system that scientifically justified human inequality and promoted injustice. His continuing influence, as exemplified by continuing citation in the medical literature, challenges the value of medical science today through its ignorance of the legacy of a person medicine continues to consider a pioneer in the field.

Otmar von Verschuer—
Human Genetics and Anthropology

A tradition of academic culture is that of honoring distinguished academics with a *Festschrift*, a celebratory volume. One person who had two *Festchrifts* published in honor of his 60th birthday was Baron Otmar von Verschuer, an internationally recognized authority in human genetics and anthropology. In June of 1939, Verschuer gave an invited lecture to the Royal Society of London.[31] In 1956, at the time the *Festschrifts* were published, he was the professor and head of the Department of Genetics at the University of Münster. One *Festchrift* was published in a German journal, *Homo*, the other in a journal of twin studies, *Acta Geneticae Medicae Gemellogiaae*, then published in Italy. The *Festschrift* in the latter journal featured an editorial honoring Verschuer as "Maestro e Esempio," master and example. It described him as:

> "A Master of clear fame and creator of men who dedicate themselves to scientific research with the spirit of a vocation, (Prof. O. V. Verschuer) is also an example of hard work and discipline for all scientists and especially for all the geneticists, beyond the confines of his School and his Nation."[32]

One of the men Verschuer helped to "create" was Josef Mengele, for whom Verschuer was professional mentor and sponsor. Mengele's Auschwitz research was financed, in part, by a research grant awarded not to Mengele, but to Verschuer. Specimens were collected from victims in Auschwitz and sent to the Kaiser-Wilhelm Institute of Anthropology in Berlin-Dahlem, then headed by Verschuer.[33-35] After the war, Verschuer was "denazified" and fined as a "fellow-traveler" and permitted to resume his professional career, which he did at Münster.[36,37] Verschuer's work continues to be cited in the scientific literature without reference to the man or the context of his work.[38]

It is through the work of such men as Rüdin and Verschuer that Nazi medicine has become part of the professional genotype of medicine today. It is through people like Rüdin, Verschuer, and Mengele that psychiatry, genetics, and twin studies have become immutably linked to the Nazi period.

We must remember that those two symbols of satanic research, Josef Mengele and Sigmund Rascher, conducted their research in order to become distinguished academics like Rüdin and Verschuer. They did not work in isolation. What we should be examining today is the academic system that created Mengele and Rascher. We should be studying how the most advanced medical scientific institutions in the world made human life dispensable; where the value of human life became secondary to that of research and academic advancement. What needs to be published and studied today is not the "scientific" data from the experiment but a recounting of the consequences of ethical compromise where human life and dignity become secondary to personal, professional, scientific, and political goals.

Conclusion

We conclude with a timeless symbol of medicine and the ethical spirit of the profession: the Greek island of Kos. In the culture of medicine, Kos symbolizes the spiritual birthplace of the profession. On Kos there exists the remains of a major temple to the Greek god of medicine, Aescelapius. Kos is the mythical birthplace of the Greek physician, Hippocrates, who created the paradigm, perhaps mythical as well, of the ethical physician. To this day, physicians make pilgrimage to Hippocrates' birthplace; many retaking the Hippocratic Oath in an ancient ceremony at the temple of Aescelapius. An oft-visited site in the town of Kos is an ancient plane tree where, legend has it, Hippocrates taught under its branches. Seeds from the plane tree of Hippocrates have been distributed around the world as part of an effort to disseminate the Hippocratic spirit.

In the summer of 1944, Kos was occupied by the German military. On July 23, the 120 Jews of Kos were assembled at the harbor, near the plane tree of Hippocrates. A small vessel arrived to pick them up, afterward joining other vessels containing the last Jews of Rhodes. From there they were transported to the Greek mainland, and from there they were conveyed by train to Auschwitz.[39]

Upon arrival at the rail siding in the Birkenau complex, the Jews of Hippocrates' birthplace were met on the ramp by the professional descendants of Hippocrates. Those licensed SS physicians who had been selected to select made a diagnosis on each of the Jews of Kos that he or she was a "useless life" and should receive the "Great Therapy of Auschwitz," which was death in "The Central Hospital" of Auschwitz. There, they all perished.

Today the island of Kos and the empty synagogue of Kos, which adjoins the plane tree of Hippocrates, symbolize the spiritual crisis of medicine arising from the Holocaust; a crisis that medicine has failed to recognize, let alone resolve.

Acknowledgments

I wish to acknowledge the guidance and assistance of Professor Michael Kater of York University (Canada). The assistance of the Israel State Archives and the Jerusalem Post is also appreciated.

Twin Research
at Auschwitz-Birkenau

Implications for the Use of Nazi Data Today

Nancy L. Segal

Introduction

Dr. Josef Mengele's medical experimentation performed at the Auschwitz-Birkenau concentration camp in Poland (1943–1945), on twins, dwarfs, and individuals with various genetic anomalies represents deplorable misuse of the twin design. Many innocent victims suffered needlessly at the hands of this cruel physician. His work and that of his collaborators has generated data regarded by medical experts as completely devoid of scientific validity. I have indicated elsewhere that on occasion, the misguided efforts of individual investigators may, unfortunately, cast shadows over the legitimate research activities of many.[1] This theme has recently been echoed by William Seidelman (this vol) in his claim that, "It is through people like Rüdin, Verschuer, and Mengele that psychiatry, genetics, and twin studies have become immutably linked to the Nazi period."

What must be done to prevent repetition of this unspeakable abuse of science by future investigators? As a psychologist with a special interest in twins and twin studies, I believe that a broad scientific perspective on twin research is requisite to considering the implications of these tragic events. Twin research is not and need not be "immutably linked" to the Nazi period if we confront the important task bequeathed to us by this unfortunate episode in human history. Difficult issues, such as: Should scientists use information derived from the concentration camps? must be seriously addressed in light of Dr. Robert Pozos' recent interest in utilizing hypothermia data collected on prisoners at Dachau.

Three areas of inquiry will be addressed. The first area reviews the basis of the classic twin design and exposes the misuse of this method by Dr. Mengele. Examples of serious methodological flaws will be cited. It will be argued that the absence of scientific validity from the twin data raises serious questions regarding the application of any data arising from Nazi medical experimentation. The second area examines the viewpoints of several twins regarding the use of Nazi data today. Excerpts of their written comments will be presented. The third area describes medical, psychological, and social issues currently confronting the Holocaust twin survivors. A review of their present situation is central to understanding their various positions on the use of Nazi data. Specific areas of concern include identification of the physical effects of the medical experiments and education of future generations about the victims' experiences in Nazi concentration camps.

Twin Methodology
and the Abuse of Twin Research

The Twin Method

Twin study methodology is central to the research programs of investigators in numerous behavioral science and medical science fields. This is because comparative analyses of similarity within genetically identical (monozygotic or MZ) twin pairs and genetically nonidentical (dizygotic or DZ) twin pairs are highly informative with respect to identifying genetic and environmental influences on human behavioral and physical traits. Greater resemblance within MZ twins, relative to DZ twins, is consistent with (although does not prove) genetic influence on the characteristic under study. Approximately 10 variants of the classic twin design are available.[2]

Twins and their families are enthusiastic research volunteers, given their interest in examining the unique biological and experiential aspects of twinship. They sincerely welcome the efforts of numerous researchers who are committed to enriching the lives of twins and contributing to knowledge about human development that can be derived from twin studies. National and local organizations of parents of twins in the US, Canada, Great Britain, and elsewhere foster research collaborations between investigators and their membership.

Dr. Josef Mengele, *Abuse of the Research Process*

The twin children of the Holocaust were the unfortunate victims of a series of very brutal and very dehumanizing experiments conducted by the infamous Auschwitz physician, Josef Mengele. Mengele's activities, conducted between the Spring, 1943 and January, 1945, included hundreds of twin pairs, although the precise figure is uncertain. The availability of 200 young male twin pairs at given times provides a sense of the large number of twin pairs involved.[3] It is estimated that 157 twins (representing both intact and nonintact twin pairs) survived. Of the 127 twins who have been identified since liberation, 121 are still alive. Searches are in progress for some twins, and several others are presumed deceased. (The names appear on the official stationery used by the organization of twin survivors.) Careful procedures were in place for locating twins on arrival at the Auschwitz-Birkenau railroad ramp. Professor Miklos Nyiszli,[4] a prisoner and forensic physican whose survival depended on assisting Dr. Mengele in many grim aspects of the twin experiments, explains:

"When the convoys arrived, soldiers scouted the ranks
lined up before box cars, hunting for twins and dwarfs.
Mothers, hoping for special treatment for their twin
children, readily gave them up to the scouts. Adult
twins, knowing that they were of interest from a scientific point of view, voluntarily presented themselves,
in the hope of better treatment." (p. 50)

January 27, 1985 marked the 40th anniversary reunion
of the liberation of Auschwitz. On this date, a group of twins
and their families traveled to Auschwitz-Birkenau to acknowledge lost relatives and to research information surrounding
their treatment in the camps. Figures 1 and 2 show twins
standing before photographs of their liberation from
Auschwitz-Birkenau, on January 27, 1945. These photographs
are part of an exhibit housed in the twins' barracks. This
event was followed by a three-day public hearing on the war
crimes of Dr. Mengele, held at Yad VaShem, in Jerusalem, Israel. Thirty twin and nontwin survivors provided public
testimony concerning the medical experimentation at
Auschwitz. This information is stored in the archives at Yad
VaShem and will, hopefully, be published in the near future.
This testimony undoubtedly comprises the most complete
record of the painful and humiliating procedures to which
the twin victims were subjected. A very brief sampling of these
procedures includes blood transfusions between twin pairs,
exposure to X-rays, extensive anthropometric measurement,
and injection of one twin with a lethal substance (e.g., typhus) for later comparison with the cotwin. Specific events
described by some victims further underline the physically
cruel and scientifically senseless nature of the experiments:
young, opposite-sex twins, one of whom was hunchbacked,
were removed from the barracks. When these children
returned, they had been stitched together back-to-back, and
were in terrible pain. Adult MZ female twins had learned
that they were to be impregnated by MZ male twins to study
the transmission of twinning. The liberation of Auschwitz,

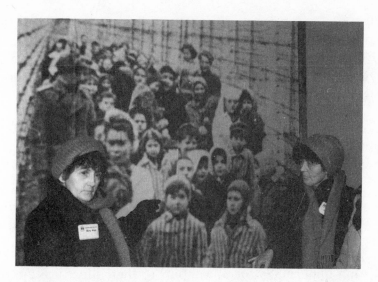

Fig. 1. Twins barracks at Birkenau, 40th Anniversary Reunion of Holocaust Twins. Identical twins, Eva Kor and Miriam Czaigher, point to their childhood photos, taken on the day of liberation from the camps, January 27, 1945. Photo credit: Dr. Nancy L. Segal.

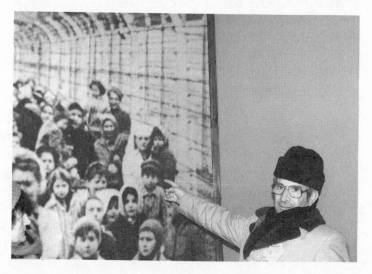

Fig. 2. Twins barracks at Birkenau, 40th Anniversary Reunion of Holocaust Twins. Morris Frankel, identical twin, points to his childhood photo, taken on the day of liberation from the camps, January 27, 1945. Photo credit: Dr. Nancy L. Segal.

fortunately, prevented this experiment from taking place. Dr. Nyiszli's eyewitness report clearly reveals that the twins of Auschwitz-Birkenau were viewed as less than human:

> "The experiments, in medical language called *in vivo*, *i.e.*, experiments performed on live human beings were far from exhausting the research possibilities in the study of twins. Full of lacunae, they offered no better than partial results. The *in vivo* experiments were succeeded by the most important phase of twin-study: the comparative examination from the viewpoints of anatomy and pathology. Here it was a question of comparing the twins' healthy organs with those functioning abnormally, or of comparing their illnesses. For that study, as for all studies of a pathological nature, corpses were needed. Since it was necessary to perform a dissection for the simultaneous evaluation of anomalies twins had to die at the same time. So it was that they met their death in the B section of one of Auschwitz's KZ barracks at the hand of Dr. Mengele. This phenomenon was unique in world medical science history." (p. 50,51)

Purpose of Twin Research
at Auschwitz-Birkenau

The motivating forces underlying Mengele's commitment to twin research remain in question. It is generally agreed that the work was intended to demonstrate a hereditary basis for group differences in behavioral and physical characteristics, a theme consistent with the Nazi biomedical vision of the superiority of the Aryan people.[6,7] In contrast, Ella Lingens, a physican at Auschwitz, indictated that Mengele's foremost concern was personal power, rather than national pride. On one occasion, he showed her some of the twin data and drawings that had been prepared by an anthropologist working with him. Her testimony at Yad VaShem underlined his fear that his precious twin data might some day fall into the hands of the Bolsheviks. It has also been suggested that the identification and application of twinning processes, for the purpose of increasing the Aryan population, were central to his research program.[6] This seems unlikely because Mengele did not systematically study the parents of twins, despite published studies (some conducted in Germany) supporting a familial component to twinning.[8]

Abuse of the Twin Method

The testimonies presented by the victims of Auschwitz were evaluated by a panel whose members represented the fields of law, history, and medical genetics.[9] The panel concluded that the medical experimentation conducted at Auschwitz was without scientific value.

"The acts of grievous bodily harm and the mutilation of the bodies and souls of the victims were perpetrated by Mengele under the guise of scientific experiments, but in truth these investigations had no apparent scientific value. Mengele's experiments were performed through coercive means upon helpless prisoners. They were part of an extensive system of pseudo-investigation conducted by Nazi medical practitioners who had violated the Hippocratic Oath."[10] (p. 2)

Reasons commonly cited to support this conclusion are summarized by Segal.[1] First, the twins were neither willing, nor informed volunteers. Second, the experiments were carried out under circumstances that were scarcely representative of the normal human condition. The debilitated physical conditions of many of the victims most certainly confounded results from the experimental procedures. Third, therapeutic reasons for applying the various medical procedures were absent. Finally, a panelist at the Yad VaShem hearing emphasized the absence of sound scientific reasoning or theory underlying the experiments. These grievous difficulties apply to the hypothermia experiments at Dachau, as well as to the twin research.

There are additional difficult aspects of the twin experiments that are less apparent than those listed above, and which further underline their dubious scientific merit. Some of these issues were raised by the twins' testimonies and have generated further inquiry.

1. Four pairs of nontwins ("pseudo-twins") have been identified. In one instance, the Nazi officers classified a pair of physically similar brothers as twins, despite their claims to the contrary. In two cases, a pair of brothers and a pair of sisters, who learned that membership in a twin pair could secure better treatment and prevent immediate death, successfully passed themselves off as twins. In a fourth case, an older twin placed in charge of a young twins' barracks "assigned" two brothers as twins in order to spare them. There may well have been other such pairs of individuals in the camps. Mengele and his staff did not, apparently, adequately verify that the participants were truly twins.

2. It is unclear if Mengele always adequately distinguished between MZ and DZ twin pairs. The most objective scientific method available for doing so is extensive serological (blood-typing) analysis, in which the blood samples of twins are compared across red blood cell systems, serum proteins, and red blood cell enzymes.[11] Lack of complete cotwin agreement for these characteristics identifies DZ twins with complete certainty. Full cotwin agreement for these characteristics identifies MZ twins with a high probability of being correct; complete certainty in the assignment of twins as MZ is precluded by occasional examples of DZ twins who share all measured blood systems in common. There are, for example, documented cases in which experienced investigators have altered classification of blood-concordant twins from MZ to DZ, based on observable differences in highly heritable traits, such as hair color or eye color.[12]

A paper reporting quantitative diversity in selected blood groups of 201 twin pairs was published by Dr. Ayres de Azevedo, a Portuguese physician at the Kaiser-Wilhelm Institute in Berlin.[13] These experiments were initiated in July, 1941 and completed in August, 1943. According to the report, the data were available from twin pairs who had participated in an earlier project directed by the Institute, during which time they had been classified as identical or fraternal by blood-typing. It was in August, 1943 that funding for Mengele's research activities at Auschwitz received approval.[6] The source of the twins and the timing of the experiments make it unlikely that de Azevedo's experiments included blood samples furnished by Mengele.[14] It is difficult to assume that blood-typing procedures were rigorously in place during Mengele's appointment at Auschwitz, especially in view of the selection procedures and the bizarre nature of the experiments. Misdiagnosis of twin pairs yields misleading estimates of genetic and environmental influence, such that careful documentation of classification procedures is requisite in current scientific publications. This problematic aspect of the twin work alone is sufficient to render the Nazi findings completely useless.

The methodological flaws in the twin experiments cast serious shadows over the hypothermia data and other data collected on nontwins by the Nazis. In particular, there is a great deal of methodological detail that is unknown and that consequently, render the data suspect (*see* Berger, this vol). This situation raises the important question: Should talented researchers invest time in determining if a questionable data set has merit? A more fruitful investment of efforts may lie in devising new and efficient means for saving lives, by means of more advanced technologies that are currently available.

Should the Data Be Used?
The Twins Speak for Themselves

The perspective of the concentration camp survivor has been strangely absent from many articles and discussions involving the use of Nazi data. It is likely that discussion of the use of the hypothermia data and related issues will continue for many generations on the part of Holocaust scholars and medical investigators. The voices of the twin survivors and other victims cannot, however, share indefinitely in this dialogue because they are growing older. It is, therefore, critical to document their attitudes and opinions at this time, in view of the public debate surrounding the use of the hypothermia data.

I mailed a brief questionnaire to 7 of the 25 twins living in the US and Canada, and to one twin living in Switzerland, for whom addresses were available. Copies of the questionnaire were also forwarded to two Israeli twins, and to Miriam Czaigher, who heads the organization of Holocaust twin survivors in Israel, for distribution to the approximately 85 twins living in that country. (Ten twins live in Australia, Rumania, Belgium, Czechoslovakia, Hungary, and West Germany.) Follow-up interviews were conducted by telephone in some cases. (Some twins found the questionnaire too upsetting to complete, but consented to be interviewed by telephone.) The questions dealt directly with the use of data gathered on twins, rather than with the hypothermia data, in order to obtain responses that were based on personal experience. One of the twins alluded to the demonstrated worthlessness of the twin data, suggesting that the questions were, therefore, not meaningful. It is important to recall, however, that much of the material collected by Mengele has never been recovered, but could possibly be located in the future. Its presence could raise the same issues now being raised in regard to the hypothermia experiments. The questionnaire is reproduced below:

1. Do you think that the medical data and other information gathered from twins at Auschwitz-Birkenau should be used by scientists or doctors today? YES NO Regardless of your answer, please give your reasons.
2. If the data are used by scientists or doctors, should the victims be acknowledged? YES NO If you answered YES, how should the victims be acknowledged?
3. Were you a victim in an experiment? YES NO

Responses from 13 twins who were victims of medical experimentation are available. They include all seven twins from the US and Canada, but only six from Israel. Nine twins were female, four twins were male, and one twin preferred to remain anonymous. The representativeness of this very modest sample is difficult to determine because the number of Israeli twins who actually received the questionnaire is uncertain. Those who did respond, however, deserve to be heard.

The twins are evenly divided between those who would and those who would not support the possible use of the twin data by physicians and scientists. Six agreed that these data should be used, whereas five argued against the use of these data. The response of one female twin was unclear; she would, however, offer herself for study if this would advance understanding of the nature and effects of the experiments. "It is very important to know," she said. One twin was uncertain as to whether or not the data should be used.

Comments provided by the twins are far more insightful than their indications of "for" or "against." This is because their statements underline the complexity of the issues surrounding the use of the Nazi data. Contradictory comments were offered by some individuals, depending on whether they approached the question on a personal or public level. It is clear, for example, that survivors from medical experimentation may have significant personal reasons for supporting study of the experimental material; some of these issues are explicated in detail in the following section. In contrast, these same individuals might not agree to the use of the data by scientists, in general.

The themes of "serving humanity" and "helping science" emerged most frequently among the responses of twins who favored the use of the data.

> "If these experiments will be of any help to humanity then I am in favor of them being used as needed."

> "I think that the data collected in experiments conducted on us should by all means be used since there were a variety of methods used and I am certain that

the data can be very beneficial to today's doctor."

"It appears that, at least in some cases, there was an attempt to induce illness by injecting bacteria and then an attempt to cure these illnesses, that is to say, we served as laboratory animals in the hands of the criminal, Mengele, and this type of research should of course be made available to the world."

Some twins underlined the importance of allowing scientists to determine what noxious substances had been injected into them 40 years ago. It may be that their interpretation of the "use of data" refers to close examination of the twins and their families to assess the effects of the experiments, rather than the use of the data in the service of humanity. Some twins suggested that if the data are used, efforts should proceed quietly, without drawing excessive public attention to their source.

In contrast, twins who did not sanction the use of the data emphasized their past and present suffering, insensitivity by the medical profession, and fear that use of the data would legitimize the Nazi research enterprise. Some among them were, however, still desperate to identify the substances they had been administered.

"No! No! No! I (we) suffered, and it is *no* 'medical data' or 'information' whatsoever!!! Scientists? Doctors? Today? When I came back NOBODY believed me! NO DOCTOR. NOBODY!! NO ONE believed me, us! And still today. Doctors? Scientists? Let them first tell us what sort of stuff they injected us with!! Let them tell me!"

"As much as I am for scientific research for the betterment of humanity, I do feel that the scientific data collected from experiments done on inmates of Nazi concentration camps should not be used. If I would agree, I feel I give a stamp of approval to the ways and means [these] experiments have been conducted and quasi-legalize it."

The fear that the Nazi data could easily fall into the wrong hands and be misused was expressed by some twins. Data from the hypothermia experiments has been used, yet how many people know the true source of these data? The fear that the use of material obtained by the Nazis might perpetuate a process in which scientists cruelly exploited individuals to secure desired information was also indicated. What is the message we wish to leave to future scientists regarding their treatment of research participants? These difficult questions escape simple solutions.

Responses to the questions of *should* and *how* victims might be acknowledged if data were used varied a great deal. They include collective acknowledgment (without identifying information), financial compensation (for suffering and for payment of current medical expenses), and newsletters to the victims. It was also suggested that the identity of the individuals responsible for the cruel experiments be preserved.

"Among the victims, there are those who were severely hurt physically and emotionally and perhaps with the best and very special care they can be helped and some of the damage can be repaired. This should be brought before the judicial committee and perhaps the government of Germany can fund this special care."

"It is imperative that the Kaiser-Wilhelm Institute be implicated as the initiator and recipient of the research data; it should not be able to get away from the ultimate responsibility for these horrors..."

Some twins would prefer not to be acknowledged.

"It is very trying for me to relive the horrors of experiments performed on me and my twin sister."

The Twins Today

Medical, Psychological, and Social Issues

Examination of the unique medical, psychological, and social issues that currently face the twin survivors enables greater understanding of their various viewpoints. The words of the surviving twins are forceful reminders that most students of the Holocaust are not victims and cannot bring the experience of continued suffering into their research efforts. Many of the twins' concerns have been previously described elsewhere,[1,15,16] so a brief survey of the major themes is presented below.

Medical Issues

A major concern facing many of the twin survivors is the possible link between experimental treatments received at Auschwitz and current medical difficulties. The twins range in age today from 47 to over 70 years of age. It is, therefore, often problematic to distinguish the effects of medical experimentation from the effects of normal aging. This dilemma is aggravated by the fact that the actual medical interventions at Auschwitz-Birkenu are often unclear. Many of the twins were, as indicated above, injected with unknown substances. This situation has made it especially difficult for some physicians to arrive at accurate diagnoses. In the case of one twin, for example, tuberculosis of the bladder was left undiagnosed for many months because it is a rare condition among middle-class populations.

Interviews and discussions with approximately 30 twins since their reunion in 1985 reveal a fierce desire to research the effects of the medical experiments. Their desire is prompted not only by concern for their own general health, but by concern for the health of their children and grandchildren.

Psychological Issues

The twins are a very unique group of child survivors. The loss of family members and the loss of the childhood years are primary among the bruises they continue to experience. Some of the twins (both from intact and nonintact pairs) who did survive were, unfortunately, unable to share their experiences for 40 years, in the mistaken belief that the other pairs of twins had perished. The establishment of CANDLES (Children of Auschwitz's Nazi Deadly Concentration Camp Survivors), in commemoration of the 40th anniversary of the liberation of Auschwitz was, therefore, a welcome opportunity to confront the past in an atmosphere of understanding and compassion.

Many of the worries and fears of the twins relate to family matters. Pregnancy was especially stressful for some women, given concerns surrounding the effects of injections on unborn children. The usual departures of children from home, for purposes of education, employment, or marriage, pose very difficult separation issues for some twins. Reunions with lost relatives are highly valued because they promise information about family histories, thus establishing links with a better past and making the present more comprehensible. For example, questions concerning familial transmission in physical characteristics, talent, and health can finally be addressed. It must be emphasized, however, that despite their pasts, the majority of twins are strong, caring people who have successfully established families and careers. The rebuilding of their lives serves as an inspiration to us all.

Elsewhere in this volume the stories of surviving twins are revealed. Their personal perspectives enable understanding of how their lives were rebuilt, and why the viewpoint of the survivor is central to debates surrounding the use of Nazi data.

Social Issues

The search for Josef Mengele and the the desire to bring him to trial was the primary goal of the twins at the time of their reunion in January, 1985. Following the reunion, government officials and the concerned public were united in their quest for the elusive physician. In June, 1985, evidence

of Mengele's death in a drowning accident in Brazil effectively halted these efforts.[3] The surviving twins, firmly convinced
that a hoax had been perpetrated, organized a meeting, "Inquest:
The Truth About Mengele," held in Terre Haute, Indiana, in
November, 1985. The purpose of this meeting was to review
the evidence together with forensic experts and representatives of the Office of Special Investigation, and to make recommendations to the appropriate authorities. A recurrent
theme was the twins' sense of neglect by the government and
medical community, as they were not included in initial evaluations of the evidence. Recently, however, new information
persuaded some individuals, such as Simon Wiesenthal (who
was previously convinced that Mengele was dead), Ben
Abraham, a Brazilian journalist, and Menahem Russek, the
Israeli Police Commissioner, that Mengele could still be
alive.[17,18] A letter to me from one of the twins (translated from
the original Hebrew) expressed their feelings most
poignantly:

> "I would like to tell you that I very much appreciate
> the meeting that you are organizing. At least there is
> someone in the big United States who is not indiffer
> ent, though sometimes it appears that everyone has
> become indifferent and they accept the fact that three
> and one-half years ago the preliminary results on the
> Mengele bones were revealed, and since then no one
> has been able to draw any final conclusions. Could
> this be? Please make sure that at the meeting you call
> for the truth to be revealed. Don't we, the little chil
> dren, the victims from Auschwitz, deserve to know the
> truth? Haven't we suffered and continue to suffer
> enough? It will be a small moral payment that will lift
> our spirits and we will know that today's world hasn't
> forgotten us. Please reveal the truth." (Mrs. Miriam
> Czaigher, March, 1989)

How do we understand that nine twins (seven of whom
participated in the Inquest), and four nontwin survivors whom
I interviewed in 1985 were not convinced of Mengele's death?

Several reasons come to mind. The twins feel the need to learn about the medical experiments and they can do so only if Mengele is alive; records that might reveal this information have never been located. Mengele is largely responsible for their life events following Auschwitz, and for this they wished to bring him to justice. In a variety of ways, the lives of the twins continue to be intimately associated with this man. Most recently, comparative analyses of blood samples from Mengele's mother and son, and DNA from bones unearthed in Brazil indicate with a high degree of certainty that Mengele is deceased. (New York Times, April 9, 1992).

The twins are fully dedicated to the purpose of educating present and future generations as to the historical events and personal stories of the Holocaust. A number of twins regularly engage in public speaking, and have made themselves available for interviews. Many of them envision the establishment of university chairs in Holocaust studies to further research and education on the origins and prevention of abuses in human research.

Closing Remarks

The conference, *"The Meaning of the Holocaust for Bioethics,"* was a direct response to a proposal by a research scientist to publish data from hypothermia experiments conducted at Dachau. The questions raised by this event and the debates that ensued, however, are universal. Additional questionable data sets have been generated by the Nazis and by other misguided investigators, and interest in their use could arise at any time. Methods for appropriately responding to the use, or proposed use, of such data must be in place.

Two themes predominated the conference: (1) Assessing the validity of the data, and (2) examining the ethics of using information gathered under inhumane circumstances. Absence of validity clearly prohibits further use of the data, but should not eliminate continued dialogue concerning the future prevention of scientific misconduct.

An informed scientific community can challenge the suspected introduction of contaminated data into the literature. A recent, excellent example is detailed in editorial communications in the *Archives of General Psychiatry.* [19-21] A paper published in that journal presented anatomical data on the brains of 13 schizophrenic patients, two of whom were twins, Ernst and Klaus H.[22] The specimens were part of the brain collection of the Vogt Institute of Brain Research in Düsseldorf, West Germany. The questionable origin of the twins' brains was exposed following presentation of the 1985 paper at the 1986 meeting of the American College of Neuropharmacology, at which time the twins' year of death (during the Nazi period) was indicated:

> "One of us (E.S.G.) told Dr. Bogerts that he and his colleagues had a responsibility to be very sure that none of the brains were the result of Nazi mass murders because such specimens would not be appropriate for medical research. Dr. Bogerts told one of us (E.S.G.) that each of the people had died a natural death, with medical records to support the cause of death. However, there were still concerns because it turned out that the two patients who had died during the Nazi period were twin brothers who died after transfer to the same hospital within several months of each other. As a German psychiatrist, one of us (M.R.H.) has a particular sensitivity to ethical issues in medical research because of the history of this period; therefore, we were both concerned."[21] (p. 774)

It was eventually determined that the deaths of the twin brothers may well have resulted from "murder through deliberate malnutrition and neglect by officials in the psychiatric hospital in which the patients were housed." Resubmission of the 1985 manuscript with the deletion of these two cases was recommended. Specific editorial guidelines for rejecting uncertain data were additionally suggested.

Recurrence of the Nazis' abuse of scientific methods and scientific research can be prevented if awareness of this period is continually maintained by faculty, students, and the public, by means of lectures, seminars, and written materials. Responsibility to our professions and to our fellow human beings dictates that this is so. The incident involving Dr. Bogerts and colleagues underlines a critical message for all investigators:

> "We believe the facts that have now been uncovered must be faced with courage and integrity as an opportunity for self-education and for the enhancement of our professional consciences."[21] (p.775,776)

Acknowledgments

I am grateful to the twin survivors who generously gave of their time to respond to the questionnaire. I also wish to thank Yosi Ben-Yanai and Steven Doyle from the University of Minnesota in Minneapolis, MN, for translation of several questionnaires and references, and Benno Müller-Hill, from the University of Cologne in West Germany, for alerting me to the paper by de Azevedo.

The Human Genome
Project in Perspective

Confronting Our Past To Protect Our Future

George J. Annas

   Nazi physicians were no historical aberration that we can easily dismiss as irrelevant to Western medicine. They drew their inspiration from many sources, including the eugenics movement in the US, and the forces that inspired them did not die with them. Others in this book have written eloquently and expertly on the history of Nazi Germany and its eugenics movement and racist policies. I have little to add here. Instead, this chapter focuses on our own medical and scientific culture, examining the forces at work in the US that we must be aware of to prevent the development of an ideology similar to that which led to the horrors perpetrated by the Nazi physicians.

   Shortly after World War II, futurists presented Western society with two views of our destiny. George Orwell, in his *1984*, saw governments akin to Germany's national socialism as taking over the world, their people forced to abide by the dictates of a totally pervasive state. Aldous Huxley, in *Brave New World*, on the other hand, thought the future would appear more benign to the citizenry. Instead of believing that they were victims of force, governments would be able to manipulate citizens, through mass media and drugs, into *wanting* to do what the state demanded. For Western countries at least, Huxley's view now seems much more likely than Orwell's. The real question, of course, is whether individuals, the state, or others will control their reproductive and personal lives.

Racism and sexism are necessary components of a repressive eugenics policy, but they are not sufficient. In Germany, it took not only a racist ideology, but a totalitarian state with the will and ability to impose this ideology ruthlessly and murderously on its people. There is no likelihood that this scenario will repeat itself in the US. On the other hand, there are powerful forces at work in our society that could combine to dramatically affect the rights and welfare of the "less than genetically perfect" and to create a culture in which people are valued (and devalued) based on their genetic endowment, and embryos screened and nurtured based on "genetic quality." Instead of an oppressive government, the forces that could bring such a result about are "all-American" ones: Our fetish for efficiency, our quest for immortality, and our belief in commercialism and its handmaiden, hype. These forces move us to want "progress" that is cost-effective (and thus, reducing the number of genetically handicapped in the population becomes an implicit goal); to seek "new" techniques that might extend our lives (thus justifying experiments on the terminally ill on the basis that they are "doomed anyway" and so have "nothing to lose"); and to oversell projects that generate large incomes for researchers, and potentially huge profits for private corporations. It seems most fruitful to explore the modern eugenics urge by examining the most ambitious genetics project in human history: The human genome project, the plan to map and sequence the human genome.

Modern Genetics in the US[1]

In Edward Albee's 1962 play, *Who's Afraid of Virginia Woolf?*, George (a historian) describes the agenda of modern biology to alter chromosomes:

...the genetic makeup of a sperm cell changed, reordered...to order, actually...for hair and eye color, stature, potency...I imagine...hairiness, features, health...and mind. Most important...Mind. All imbalances will be corrected, sifted out...propensity for various diseases will be gone, longevity assured. We will have a race of men...test-tube-bred...incubatorborn...superb and sublime.

George's view of the future was sinister and threatening in the early 1960s. Today these same sentiments seem almost quaint. Mapping and sequencing the estimated three billion base pairs of the human genome (the 50,000–100,000 genes that make up the 22 autosomal chromosome haploid set and the two sex chromosomes) is "in;" raising serious questions about the project itself is "out." There is money to be made here, and even the ethicists are slated to have their share.

The *Wall Street Journal* summarized the case for the human genome project in early 1989 when it editorialized, "The techniques of gene identification, separation and splicing now allow us to discover the basic causes of ailments and, thus, to progress toward cures and even precursory treatments that might ward off the onset of illness ranging from cancer to heart disease and AIDS." All that is lacking "is a blueprint—a map of the human genome." Noting that some members of the European Parliament had suggested that ethical questions regarding eugenics should be answered "*before it proceeds*," the *Journal* opined, "This, of course, is a formula for making no progress at all." The editorial concluded, "The Human Genome Initiative...may well invite attack from those who are fearful of or hostile to the future. It should also attract the active support of those willing to *defend the future*."[2]

The National Institutes of Health (NIH) created a National Center for Human Genome Research, which funds proposals to study "the ethical, social and legal issues that may arise from the application of knowledge gained as a result" of the human genome project. The original announcement was rather vague, but made clear that such projects are to be about the "immense potential benefit to humankind" of the project, and focus on "the best way to ensure that the information is used in the most beneficial and responsible manner." Those with less optimism apparently need not apply. Later announcements were more detailed, but still upbeat on the project's beneficial potential.[3]

James Watson is the head of the Center. He is perhaps the genome project's leading cheerleader, having said, among other things, that the project provides "an extraordinary potential for human betterment...We can have at our disposal the ultimate tool for understanding ourselves at the molecular level...The time to act is now." And, "How can we not do it? We used to think our fate is in our stars. Now we know, in large measure, our fate is in our genes."[4] And more recently, "A more important set of instruction books will never be found in human beings."[5]

Are there any difficult legal and ethical problems involved in mapping the human genome, or is everything as straightforward and rosy as its advocates paint it? NIH plans to devote 1–3% or more of its genome budget to exploring social, legal, and ethical issues. Although any serious attention to these issues by scientists is virtually unprecedented, this commitment remains trivial. James Watson sees few dangers ahead. But Watson himself, reflecting on his own early career, wrote in 1967: "Science seldom proceeds in the straightforward, logical manner...its steps are often very human events in which personalities and cultural traditions play major roles."[6]

Predicting the Future

The human genome project has been frequently compared to both the Manhattan Project and the Apollo Project, and "big biology" seems ecstatic to have its own megaproject of a size formerly restricted to physicists and engineers. But the sheer size of these two other projects obscures more important lessons. The Manhattan Project is familiar, but it still teaches us volumes about science and the unforeseen impact of technological "advance." In late 1945, Robert Oppenheimer testified on the role of science in the development of the atomic bomb before the US Congress:

> When you come right down to it, the reason that we did this job is because it was an organic necessity. If you are a scientist, You cannot stop such a thing. If you are a scientist, you believe that it is good to find out how the world works; that it is good to find what the realities are; that it is good to turn over to mankind at large the greatest possible power to control the world...[7]

What is striking in Oppenheimer's testimony is his emphasis on the notion that science is unstoppable with the simultaneous insistence that its goal is *control* over nature, irreconcilable concepts that seem equally at the heart of the human genome project. Of course, with the atomic bomb, control quickly became illusory. The bomb, which carries with it the promise of the total annihilation of humankind, has made the nation state ultimately unstable and at the mercy of every other nation with the bomb. Necessity has forced all nuclear powers to move, however slowly, from mutually assured destruction (MAD) toward a transnational community.

The Apollo Project had its own problems. An engineering exercise, it was about neither the inevitability of scientific advance nor the control of nature. Instead, it was about military advantage and commercialism, disguised as science and hyped as a peace mission. As Walter McDougall has persuasively documented, the plaque Astronaut Paul Armstrong left on the moon that read, "We came in peace for all mankind," was ironic:

> The moon was not what space was all about. It was about science, sometimes spectacular science, but mostly about spy satellites, and comsats, and other orbital systems for military and commercial advantage. "Space for peace" could no more be engineered than social harmony, and the UN Outer Space

Treaty...drew many nations into the hunt for advantage, not integration, through spaceflight.[8]

The *Wall Street Journal* seems more attuned to the commercial applications of gene mapping and sequencing than NIH, and Congressional support of the project is based primarily on the hope that mapping the genome can help the US maintain its lead over Japan in the biotechnology industry. Neither ethicists nor social planners played any real role in either the Manhattan or Apollo Projects. It appears they will at least play some minor role in the Genome Project. What should the role be, and how should it be structured?

The Legal and Ethical Issues[9]

To oversimplify somewhat, there are three levels of issues raised by the Human Genome Project: individual/family; society; and species.

Level One (Individual/Family) Issues

Genetic screening and counseling are techniques that have been in widespread use in the US for more than two decades. Since we have had a number of large-scale genetic screening and counseling programs, including Tay-Sachs, sickle cell disease, and neural tube defects, it might be supposed that we have solved the major social policy issues raised by such screening. This would be incorrect. Partly this is owing to the fact that each genetic disease has unique characteristics, and thus poses some unique issues. For example, some diseases occur most frequently in specific racial or ethnic groups, raising potential issues of discrimination and stigmatization. Other screening tests, such as those for neural tube defects, can only be done on pregnant women, and abortion is the only "treatment." Still others can only be performed on newborns, and newborn screening for conditions, such as phenylketonuria (PKU), that require immediate treatment to prevent harm, has been made mandatory by almost all states.

Even though we have not solved any of the major issues raised by past genetic screening and counseling cases, we have been able to identify the major factors to be considered before initiating a screening program:

1. The frequency and severity of the condition;
2. The availability of treatment of documented efficacy;
3. The extent of which detection by screening improves the outcome;
4. The validity and safety of the screening tests;
5. The adequacy of resources to assure effective screening and counseling follow-up;
6. The costs of the program; and
7. The acceptance of the screening program by the commu-nity, including both physicians and the public.

This list primarily relates to the scientific validity and a cost/benefit analysis of the testing procedure. In addition, two major legal issues are implicit in all genetic screening programs: autonomy and confidentiality. Autonomy requires that all screening programs be voluntary, and that consent to them is sought only after full information concerning the implications of a positive finding is disclosed and understood. Confidentiality requires that the results not be disclosed to anyone else without the individual's consent.

Provided that testing remains voluntary, and that the results are only disclosed with the individual's permission, genetic testing based on one's genome raises questions only of degree rather than kind. The degree is that instead of one or scores of conditions that can be screened for, there may be hundreds or even thousands. Perhaps even more importantly, we may find that certain genes predispose a person to specific illnesses, such as breast cancer or Alzheimer's disease. This information may be very troubling to individuals, and will be of great interest to health insurance companies and employers.[10]

We have so far managed to develop genetic screening and counseling as tools that we have permitted individuals and families to use or not use as they see fit. This has followed the "medical model" of the beneficent doctor–patient relationship: A model of mutual consent in which decisions are made for benefit of the patient. This model has served us well to date in expanding the reproductive options of individuals. Level Two concerns move us away from concern with the individual, to concern with society itself.

Level Two (Societal) Issues

Societal issues involved in the genome cluster around three areas: population-based screening, resource allocation and commercialism, and eugenics. Of these the first overlaps Level One concerns (since population screening can be used to identify individuals to help them); the last two areas are more uniquely "societal."

The issue of resource allocation itself has at least three aspects. The first is the obvious one: What percentage of the nation's research budget should be devoted to the Human Genome Project? Answering this question requires us to consider how research priorities are set in science and who should set them. With the federal government making a major commitment to this program (currently approximately $100 million annually to NIH and US Department of Energy), should Congress appropriate funds directly to the genome project (as it is currently doing) or should the program compete directly with other proposed research projects, and be peer-reviewed?

The second aspect involves making the fruits of the genome project available to all those who want them. This involves at least two questions. The first is the issue of commercialism, and who owns and can patent the products that are produced by the genome project. Should individual companies and scientists be able to patent or copyright maps and sequences of specific areas of human genome in order to encourage them to become involved in mapping research? The other issue can be summed up in three words: National health insurance, i.e., should the genetic tests and their follow-up procedures be made part of a "minimum benefit package" under national health insurance (or some other scheme for universal access), or should they only be available to those who can pay for them privately?

A third aspect of the resource allocation issue is probably the most intrinsically interesting. It involves determining resource priorities between spending on identifying and treating genetic diseases, as opposed to spending directly to correct other conditions that cause disease, such as poverty, drug and alcohol addiction, lack of housing, poor education, and lack of access to decent medical care. What is the social impact of putting the spotlight on a project like the Human Genome Project? Could the fact that we are vigorously pur-suing this project lead us to downplay environmental pollution, worksite hazards, and other major social problems that cause disease based on the hope that we will someday find a "genetic fix" to permit humans to "cope" with these healthy conditions?

The third Level Two issue, and the most relevant one to this book, is the issue of eugenics. This issue is perhaps the most difficult to address because of the highly emotional reaction many individuals have when one mentions the racist genocide of the Nazis, that was based on a eugenic program founded on a theory of "racial hygiene."[11] Although repugnant, the Nazi experience and legacy demands careful study to determine what led to it, why scientists and physicians supported it and collaborated in developing its theory and making possible its execution, and how it was implemented by a totalitarian state. In this regard our own national experience with racism, sterilization, and immigration quotas must be reexamined. In so doing, we are likely to rediscover the powerful role of economics in driving our own views of evolution (in the form of social Darwinism) and who should propagate.

The US Supreme Court, for example, wrote in 1927, with clear reference to World War I, that eugenics by involuntary sterilization of the mentally retarded was constitutionally acceptable based on utilitarianism:

> We have seen more than once that the public welfare may call upon the best citizens for their lives. It would be strange if it could not call upon those who already sap the strength of the State for these lesser sacri-

fices often not felt to be such by those concerned, in order to prevent our being swamped with incompetence. It is better for all the world, if instead of waiting to execute degenerate offspring for crime, or to let them starve for their imbecility, society can prevent those who are manifestly unfit from continuing their kind.[12]

Oliver Wendell Holmes' rhetoric may seem ancient history, but in 1988, the US Congress' Office of Technology Assessment (OTA), in discussing the "Social and Ethical Considerations" raised by the Human Genome Project, developed a similar theme:

Human mating that proceeds without the use of genetic data about the risks of transmitting diseases will produce greater mortality and medical costs than if carriers of potentially deleterious genes are alerted to their status and encouraged to mate with noncarriers or to use artificial insemination or other reproductive strategies.[13]

The likely primary reproductive strategy, mentioned only in passing in the report, will be genetic screening of human embryos, already technically feasible, but not nearly to the extent possible once the genome is understood. Such screening need not be required; people will want it, even insist on it as their right. As OTA notes, "New technologies for identifying traits and altering genes make it possible for eugenic goals to be achieved through technological as opposed to social control."[14] Huxley's *Brave New World,* rather than Orwell's *1984,* seems to be in our future.

It would be comforting to be able to conclude that our connection with medicine's Nazi past is only theoretical, and that no direct links can be shown. Unfortunately, recent scholarship has dramatically demonstrated that it is impossible to conceal linkages between even a project as highly touted and visible as the Human Genome Project, and the horrors of Nazi "experimentation" in the concentration camps. By almost any measurement, Dr. Josef Mengele, the "Angel of Death," was one of the most notorious of the Nazi physicians. He was able to escape to South America after the war, and was never brought to justice. Nonetheless, an indictment was drawn up listing many of his crimes, and sworn testimony was recorded. This and other eyewitness accounts summarize the cold brutality of this M.D.-Ph.D. "man of science." Some of his most horrifying work involved genetically related experiments performed on children who were twins, many of whom he personally murdered. In an affidavit, one of his prison assistants, Dr. Miklos Nyiszli, describes how Mengele once killed 14 Gypsy twins himself:

> In the work room next to the dissecting room, fourteen Gypsy twins were waiting and crying bitterly. Dr. Mengele didn't say a single word to us, and prepared a 10 cc and a 5 cc syringe. From a box he took Evipal and from another box he took chloroform, which was in 20 cc glass containers, and put these on the operating table. After that the first twin was brought in...a fourteen year old girl. Dr. Mengele ordered me to undress the girl and put her head on the dissecting table. The he injected the Evipal into her right arm intravenously. After the child had fallen asleep, he felt for the left ventricle of the heart and injected 10 cc of chloroform. After one little twitch the child was dead, whereupon Dr. Mengele had her taken into the corpse chamber. In this manner all fourteen twins were killed during the night.[15]

Dr. Nyiszli first observed this method of killing when it was used on four pairs of twins all under 10 years of age. Mengele was interested in them because three of the pairs had different colored eyes. He had them killed, and their eyes and other organs removed and shipped to Professor Otmar Von Verschuer of the Kaiser Wilhem Institute in Berlin, marked "War Materials-Urgent."[16]

What do Mengele's experiments have to do with the Human Genome Project? Nothing directly, but the indirect linkages are disturbing and attest to our ability to look the

other way to avoid unpleasant associations. Robert Jay
Lifton[17] and Benno Muller-Hilll[18] have both documented
Mengele's relationship to Otmar Von Verschuer. Von Verschuer
was Mengele's professor in the late 1930s, introduced him to
twin research with its racial implications (Von Verschur was
interested in whether one could purify a factor that made
one race less susceptible to disease than another, and use
it to protect the members of the other race), and personally
obtained funding and approval from the German government
for Mengele's "research" on twins at Auschwitz. Mengele
regularly sent his "results" and specimens to Von
Verschuer, and was highly regarded by him. As Von
Verschuer put it himself to the German Research Association:

> My assistant Dr. med. and Dr. phil. Mengele has joined
> as a collaborator in this research [using serum pro-
> teins from one race to protect another race from infec-
> tious diseases]. He is an SS officer and camp doctor in
> the concentration camp Auschwitz. Anthropological
> work is in progress and blood samples are being sent
> to my laboratory with the approval of the Reichsfuhrer
> SS [Himmler].[19]

The link between Mengele and Verschuer is not in doubt.
But it took Dr. William E. Seidelman to link Verschuer with
modern genetics in the US, and thus with the Human
Genome Project itself. As Seidelman noted in 1988,[20] Victor McKusick had cited Von Verschuer's genetics work in a
1982 article on mapping the human genome in which
Verschuer was implicitly given credit for doing the first studies to identify genetic loci for specific traits "mainly by
mendelizing phenotypes."[21] Always a leader in the Human
Genome Project, McKusick later became the head of the
international genome organization, the Human Genome
Organization (HUGO), and is currently the chairman of its
ethics committee. McKusick had no idea that he was citing
the work of the sponsor of one of the most notorious Nazi
physician genetics experimenters. But that is the point: The

Human Genome Project, and all modern genetics, can be inadvertently infected with the Nazi doctor virus. It is our duty to recognize this infection and treat it before it spreads.

Level Three (Species) Issues[22]

Level Three issues relate to the fact that powerful new technologies do not just change what human beings can do, they change the way we think, especially about ourselves. In this respect, maps may become particularly powerful thought transformers. Maps model reality to help us understand it. Columbus changed the shape of the world's map forever; from a flat chart to a spherical globe. Copernicus and Vesalius published their great works in the same year, 1543. *On the Motions of Heavenly Bodies* made it clear that the earth rotated around the sun, not the other way around. The earth could no longer be seen as the "center" of the universe.

Vesalius' "maps" of the human anatomy may have been even more important metaphors for us, for in dissecting the human body, Vesalius insisted that human beings could nonetheless only be understood as whole beings: rather than as parts that can be fitted together to manufacture life forms. For Vesalius, who shows 21 of 73 drawings in his *Fabrica* as full figured humans, and 10 of 12 drawings in his *Epitome* as full figured humans, the emphasis is firmly on the person, even though the treatise is concerned with the person's body parts. This is in stark contrast to the bar graph illustrations used by contemporary geneticists in "mapping" the genome, which are totally devoid of human reference, almost life without life. Does this reconceptualization of the human with a new "map" encourage us to travel into areas that could lead us to simultaneously misunderstand and demean what it is to be human?

What new human perspectives, or what new perspectives on humans, will a sequential map of the three billion base pairs of the human genome bring? The most obvious is that breaking "human beings" down into six billion "parts" is the ultimate in reductionism. James Watson, as already

noted, has used such reductionist language in promoting the
Human Genome Project, noting "our fate is in our genes."
Such a view suggests most of the Level Three concerns.

The first is the consequence of viewing humans as an
assemblage of molecules, arranged in a certain way. The
almost inevitable tendency in such a view is that expressed
in *Brave New World*. People could view themselves and each
other as products that can be "manufactured," and subject to
quality control measures. People could be "made to measure,"
both literally and figuratively. If people are so seen, we might
not only try to manipulate them as embryos and fetuses, but
we might also see the resulting children as products themselves. This raises the current stakes in the debates about
frozen embryos and surrogate mothers to a new height: If
children are seen as products, the purchase and sale of the
resulting children themselves, not only sperm, ova, and
embryos, may be seen as reasonable.

Second, to the extent that genes are considered more
important than environment, our actions may be viewed as
genetically determined, rather than as a result of free will.
Genetic predispositions are likely to be used in education, and
perhaps job placement and military assignments. For
example, if mathematical ability is found to be genetic, it
will be difficult for schools to resist using this information to
track, grade, and promote the "genetically gifted" in math classes.

Finally, we know that diseases and abnormalities are
social constructs as well as facts of nature. Myopia, for
example, is well accepted; whereas obesity is not. We won't
discover a completely "normal" or "standard" human genome,
but we may invent one. If we do, what variation will society
view as permissible before an individual's genome is labeled
"substandard" or "abnormal"? And what impact will such a
construct of genetic normalcy have on society and on "substandard" individuals? For example, what variation in a
fetus should prompt a couple to opt for abortion, or a genetic
counselor to suggest abortion? What variation should prompt
a counselor to suggest sterilization? What interventions will
society deem acceptable in an individual's life based on his

or her genetic composition? Should health care insurance companies, for example, be able to disclaim financial responsibility for the medical needs of a child whose parents knew prior to conception or birth that the child would be born with seriously "abnormal" genome? Should employers be able to screen out workers on the basis of their genomes? These and many other similar issues exist today based on screening for single site genes. But the magnitude of the screening possibilities that may result from analysis of the map of the human genome will raise these issues to new heights, and will almost inevitably change the way we think about ourselves and what it means to be human.

Policy Options

What options exist for policy makers who would like to have the benefits of the human genome project and minimize or control the potential harms? At a Workshop on International Cooperation for the Human Genome Project held in Valencia in October, 1988, French researcher Jean Dausset argued that the genome project posed great potential hazards that could open the door to Nazi-like atrocities. To attempt to avoid such results, he suggested that the conferees agree on a moratorium on genetic manipulation of germ line cells, and a ban on gene transfer experiments in early embryos. Reportedly, the proposal won wide agreement among the participants, and was watered down to a resolution calling for "international cooperation" only after American participant Norton Zinder successfully argued that the group had no authority to make such a resolution stick.[23]

Zinder was correct. A moratorium and ban on research that no one wants to do at this point would have only symbolic value, and negative symbolic value at that. It would signal that the scientists could handle the ethical issues alone, and could monitor their own work. It would tend to quiet the discussion of both germ line research and gene transfers in early embryos—both subjects that deserve wide public debate. But Dausset also had a point. The Nazi atrocities grew out of the combination of a public health ethic that

saw the abnormal as disposable, and a tyrannical dictatorship
that was able to give physicians and public health officials
unlimited authority to put their program into bestial practice.

Ethics is generally taken seriously by physicians and
scientists only when it either fosters their agenda or does
not interfere with it. If it cautions a slower pace or a more
deliberate consideration of science's darker side, it is dismissed as "fearful of the future," anti-intellectual, or simply
uninformed. The Human Genome Project has already been
overhyped and oversold. It is the obligation of those who take
our future seriously to insure that the personal, societal, and
species dangers, as well as the commercial and medical
opportunities, are rigorously and publicly explored. We must
get beyond Honey's response to George's musings on our
genetic future in Albee's play: "How exciting!"

Our own "brave new world" will not be ruled by scientists, any more than scientists decided whether to use the
atomic bomb, or whether to send a man to the moon. Social
policy will ultimately be set by elected politicians and their
advisers. It is already past time to begin to involve the elec-
torate in a national debate about the appropriate uses of the
products of the Human Genome Project. In this discussion,
the focus should be on two central questions: What does it
mean to be human? And how can human life on this planet
be enhanced?

With both real and psychological walls crumbling around
the world, the time may be at hand for meaningful international dialogue and cooperation on the Human Genome
Project. It may also be possible, although perhaps this is
wishful thinking, to engage the world in a responsible debate
about all of our futures, and to do so in a manner that strives
to enhance the dignity of all human beings. Playwright,
former political prisoner, and current president of Czechoslovakia, Vaclav Havel expressed it well in a 1984 speech on
"Politics and Conscience:"

> To me the smokestack soiling the heavens is...the symbol
> of an age which seeks to transcend the boundaries of
> the natural world and its norms and to make the mat-

ter merely a private concern, a matter of subjective preference and private feeling. The process of anonymisation and depersonalization of power, and its reduction to a mere technology of rule and manipulation, has a thousand masks...States grow ever more machine-like, men are transformed into casts of extras, as voters, producers, consumers, patients, tourists or soldiers....If we can defend our humanity, then, perhaps, there is a hope of sorts that we shall also find some more meaningful ways of balancing our natural claims to shared economic control, to dignified social status...As long, however, as our humanity remains defenseless, we will not be saved by any better economic functioning, just as no filter on a factory smokestack will prevent the general dehumanization. To what purpose a system functions is, after all, more important than how it does so; might it not function quite smoothly, after all, in the service of total destruction?...[24]

Havel then adds that our task must be to resist "at every step and everywhere, the irrational momentum of anonymous, impersonal and inhuman power—the power of ideologies, systems, apparat, bureaucracy, artificial languages and slogans...whether it takes the form of consumption, advertising, repression, technology, or cliche...We must not be ashamed that we are capable of love, friendship, solidarity, sympathy and tolerance, but just the opposite: We must set these fundamental dimensions of our humanity free from their 'private' exile and accept them as the only genuine starting point of meaningful human community."[25] In Havel's view, machine-men become alienated even from themselves; and technology cannot save them from artificiality; only their "natural" humanness and their ability to distinguish good from evil can save humankind from itself.

Havel obviously did not have the Human Genome Project in mind when he delivered his 1984 speech, nor when he delivered a speech to a joint session of the US Congress in February, 1990. Nonetheless, his 1984 words aptly summarize the challenge we face, and his 1990 words to Con-

gress properly insist that we all take personal responsibility
for our own actions and the future of our world:

> Without a global revolution in the sphere of human
> consciousness, nothing will change for the better in the
> sphere of our being...We still don't know how to put
> morality ahead of politics, science and economy. We
> are still incapable of understanding that the only genu-
> ine backbone of all our actions, if they are to be moral,
> is responsibility—responsibility to something higher
> than my family, my country, my company, my success.[26]

There is, of course, some artificiality in linking Nazi
eugenics with contemporary genome research, just as
Robert Jay Lifton and Eric Markusen found some artificiality in
linking the genocidal mentality of the Nazis with the genocidal
mentality of the nuclear weapons advocates. Nonetheless,
the similarities may be ultimately more important than the
differences in helping us to understand our own relationship to humankind's ability to annihilate itself with nuclear
weapons. We will not physically destroy humankind with
genetic "advances," but we cannot begin to understand their
implications without understanding our past uses and mis-
uses of eugenics. Drawing on the Holocaust, Lifton and
Markusen help tie together the Nazi horrors, the Human
Genome Project, and the eloquence of Havel, while consciously referring only to the first. Noting that " 'existence as
such' is inseparable from survival of the human species," they
argue that we must realign our self-concern to encompass
concern about all humankind:

> ...the species self is likely to advocate moral and po-
> litical policies attuned not to only a single group or
> nation but to all humankind. Only by so doing can we
> take in and experience larger human realities of threat
> and suffering and resist numbing and brutalization.
> We can then speak of a continuous mutual strength-
> ening of species consciousness and species self on the
> one hand, and confrontation of genocide and genocide
> threat on the other.[27]

To paraphrase Havel, Lifton, and Markusen: Only by using our species sense can we confront the brutality of our eugenic past and thereby strengthen our ability to resist the anonymizing threats of the new genetics to our personhood and our humanity.

Bibliography

Alexander, L. (1946) *The Treatment of Shock from Prolonged Exposure to Cold, Especially in Water.* (US Department of Commerce, Washington DC).

Alexander, L. (1948) War crimes, their social-psychological aspects. *Am. J. Psychiatry* **105**, 170–177.

Alexander, L. (1949) Medical science under dictatorship. *N. Engl. J. Med.* **241**, 39–47.

Alexander, L. (1966) Limitations of experimentation on human beings with special reference to psychiatric patients. *Dis. Nerv. Syst.* **27**, 61–65.

Almog, S. (1988) *Anti-Semitism Through the Ages* (Pergamon Press, New York).

Altman, L. K. (1990, May 17) Nazi data on hypothermia termed unscientific. *New York Times,* B11.

Aly, G. and Roth, K. H. (1984) The legalization of mercy killings in medical and nursing institutions in Nazy Germany from 1938–1941. *Int. J. Law Psychiatry* **7**, 145–163.

Amir, A. (1977) *Euthanasia in Nazi Germany.* Ph.D Dissertation, SUNY, Albany.

Anderson, J. (1984) The twins of Auschwitz today. *Parade* pp. 3-7.

Angell, M. (1990) The Nazi hypothermia experiments and unethical research today. *N. Engl. J. Med.* **322**, 1462–1462.

Annas, G. and Grodin, M., eds. (1992) *The Nazi Doctors and the Nuremberg Code* (Oxford University Press, New York).

Anonymous (1988) Phosgene data stir anger. *Chem. Marketing Rep.* **233(13)**, 5,14.

Arad, Y., Gutmann, Y., and Margaliot, A., eds., (1985) *Documents on the Holocaust* (Pergamon Press, New York).

Arendt, H. (1987) *Eichmann in Jerusalem: A Report in the Banality of Evil* (Penguin Books, New York).

Arthur, R. J., Friedmann, C. T. H., and Faguet, R. A. (1982) *Psychiatric Syndromes in Prisoners of War and Concentration Camp Survivors. Extraordinary Disorders of Human Behavior. Critical Issues in Psychiatry* (Plenum Press, New York).

Ascherson, A. (1987) The death doctors. *NY Rev. Books* **28**, 29–33.

Aziz, P. (1976) *Doctors of Death* (Ferni Publishers, Geneva).

Baader, G. and Schultz, U., eds., (1980) *Medizin und Nationalsozialismus* (Verlagsgesellschaft Gesundheit, West Berlin).

Baker, S. (1985) Nazi science. *Omni* **7**, p. 31.

Bauer, Y., ed. (1989) *Remembering for the Future* (Pergamon Press, New York).

Bayle, F. (1950) *Croix Gammée Contre Caducée* (Neustadt, Centre de l'imprimene Nationale).

Beecher, H. K. (1966) Ethics and clinical research. *N. Engl. J. Med.* **274**, 1354–1360.

Beecher, H. K. (1970) *Research and the Individual* (Little Brown, Boston).

Berben, P. (1975) The Medical Experiments. *Dachau: 1933–1945, The Official History* (Norfolk Press, London), pp. 123–137.

Berger, R. L. (1990) Nazi science—The Dachau hypothermia experiments. *N. Engl. J. Med.* **322(20)**, 1435–1440.

Beyerchen, A. D. (1977) *Scientists Under Hitler* (Yale University Press, New Haven, CT).

Biagioli, M. (1992) Science, modernity and the final solution, in *Probing the Limits of Representation* (Friedlander, S., ed.), Harvard University Press, Cambridge, MA.

Bloch, F. (1986) Medical scientists in the Nazi era. *Lancet* **315**, p. 375.

Bock, G. (1986) *Zwangssterilisation im Nationalsozialismus* (Westdeutscher Verlag, Opladen).

Bogerts, B. (1988) The brains of the Vogt collection. *Arch. Gen. Psychiatry* **45**, 774.

Boozer, J. S. (1980) Children of Hippocrates: Doctors in Nazi Germany. *Ann. Am. Acad. Pol. Soc. Sci.* **435**, 83–97.

Brackman, A. C. (1987) *The Other Nuremberg* (Morrow, New York).

Brieger, G. (1978) History of human experimentation, in *Encyclopedia of Bioethics* (Reich, W. T., ed.), Free Press, New York, **2**, 683–692.

Browning, C. (1988) Genocide and public health: German doctors and Polish Jews. *Holocaust Genocide Stud.* **3(1)**, 21–36.

Burleigh, M. and Wipperman, W. (1992) *The Racial State: Germany 1933–1945* (Cambridge University Press, New York).

Caplan, A. L. (1988) *Data Too Tainted With Horror to Be of Use* (St. Paul Pioneer Press, St. Paul, MN).

Caplan, A. L. (1989) *Bury But Study This Sad Legacy* (St. Paul Pioneer Press, St. Paul, MN).

Caplan, A. L. (1989) The Meaning of the Holocaust for Bioethics. *Hastings Cent. Rep.* **19,4:** 2,3.

Caplan, A. (1990) The end of a myth. *Dimensions: J. Holocaust Stud.* **5,2**, 13–18.

Caplan, A. L. (1990) Telling it like it was. *Hastings Cent. Rep.* **March/ April,** 47,48.

Cohen, A. (1974) Animal experimentation. *J. Halacha Contemp. Soc.* **6,** pp. 19–32.

Cohen, B. (1989) Ethics of using medical data from Nazi experiments. *Midstream* **35,5,** pp. 1–5.

Cohen, C. (1983) 'Quality of Life' and the analogy with the Nazis. *J. Med. Philos.* **8 (2),** 113–135.

Anonymous (1989) Contemporary lessons from Nazi medicine. *IME Bull.* **47,** 13–20.

Curran, W. J. (1986) The forensic investigation of the death of Josef Mengele. *N. Engl. J. Med.* **315(17),** 1071–1073.

Dadrian, V. N. (1986) The role of Turkish physicians in the World War I genocide of Ottoman Armenians. *Holocaust Genocide Stud.* **1(2),** 169–192.

Davis, H. (1985) Angels of life. *Hadassah* 21–24.

Dawidowicz, L. *The Holocaust and the Historians* (Harvard University Press, Cambridge, MA).

Dawidowicz, L. (1975) *The War Against the Jews, 1933–1945* (Holt, Rinehart and Winston, New York).

Degener, T. (1990) Debates across social movements on reproductive technologies, genetic engineering and eugenics, in *Ethical Issues in Disability and Rehabilitation* (Duncan, B. and Woods, D. E., eds.), World Rehabilitation Fund, New York, pp. 73–82.

Dickman, S. (1989) Scandal over Nazi victims' corpses rocks universities. *Nature* **337,** p. 195.

Dicks, H. (1972) *Licensed Mass Murder* (Basic Books, New York).

Dixon, B. (1985) Citations of shame; Scientists are still trading on Nazi atrocities. *New Scientist* **105,** pp. 410–412.

Duncan, P. (1980) Martyr or murderer? The role of Wolfram Sievers on the Nazi criminal medical experiments. *Red River Valley Hist. J. World Hist.* **4(3),** 243–268.

Einspruch, B. (1989) Racial hygiene. *JAMA* **261,** p. 300.

Fackenheim, E. L. (1986) Concerning authentic and unauthentic responses to the Holocaust. *Holocaust Genocide Stud.* **1(1),** 101–120.

Fahrenkrug, W. H. (1987) Conceptualization and management of alcohol-related problems in Nazi Germany, 1933–45, in *The Social History of Alcohol* (Barrows, S., Room, R., and Verhey, J., eds.), University Press, Berkeley, CA.

Freedman, B. (1975) A moral theory of consent. *Hastings Cent. Rep.*

Freedman, M. H. (1985) Nazi research: Too evil to cite. *Hastings Cent. Rep.,* **August,** 31,32.

Freund, P. (1969) Legal frameworks for human experimentation. *Daedalus* **248,** 319–330.

Freund, P., ed. (1972) *Experimentation With Human Subjects* (George Allen & Unwin, London).

Gallagher, H. G. (1990) *By Trust Betrayed: Patients and Physicians in the Third Reich* (Henry Holt, New York).

Gilbert, M. (1988) *Atlas of the Holocaust* (Pergamon Press, Elmsford, NY).

Glass, B. (1989) The roots of Nazi eugenics. *Q. Rev. Biol.* **64(2),** 175–180.

Golby, S. (1971) Experiments at the Willowbrook State School. *Lancet* **1,** p. 749.

Graham, L. R. (1977) Science and values: The eugenics movement in Germany and Russia in the 1920s. *Am. Hist. Rev.* **82 (5),** 1133–1164.

Haas, A. (1988) Ethics where there are none: A Holocaust survivor remembers. *NYU Physician* **34,** 61–67.

Hallic, P. (1979) *Lest Innocent Blood Be Shed* (Harper, New York).

Hanauske-Abel, H. (1986) From nazi holocaust to nuclear holocaust: A lesson to learn? *Lancet* **8501(2),** 271–273.

Hastings Center (1976) *Biomedical Ethics and the Shadow of Nazism,* Special Supplement.

Hilberg, R. (1985) *The Destruction of the European Jews* (Holmes & Meir, New York).

Hoenig, L. J. (1985) Nazi research: Too evil to cite. *Hastings Cent. Rep.* **August,** 31,32.

Howard-Jones, N. (1982) Human experimentation in historical and ethical perspective. *Soc. Sci. Med.* **16,** 1429–1448.

Hubbard, R. (1986) Eugenics and prenatal testing. *Int. J. Health Serv.* **16(2),** 227–242.

Ingelfinger, F. J. (1972) Informed (but uneducated) consent. *N. Engl. J. Med.* **287(9),** 465,466.

Ivy, A. C. (1947) Nazi war crimes of a medical nature. *Fed. Bull.* **33,** 267–272.

Ivy, A. C. (1948) The history and ethics of the use of human subjects in medical experiments. *Science* **108,** 1–5.

Jakobovits, I. (1975) *Jewish Medical Ethics* (Bloch, New York).

Jonas, H. (1980) Philosophical reflections on experimenting with human subjects, in *Philosophical Essays: From Current Creed to Technological Man* (University of Chicago, Chicago, IL), 105–131.

Kak, J. (1972) *Experimentation with Human Beings* (Russell Sage Foundation, New York).

Kampe, N. (1987) Normalizing the Holocaust? The recent historians' debate in the Federal Republic of Germany. *Holocaust Genocide Stud.* **2(1),** 61–80.

Kater, M. (1986) Physicians in crisis at the end of the Weimar Republic, in *Unemployment and the Great Depression in Weimar, Germany* (Staachura, P., ed.), Macmillan, Basingstoke, pp. 49–77.

Kater, M. H. (1987) The burden of the past: Problems of a modern historiography of physicians and medicine in Nazi Germany. *German Stud. Rev.* **10**, 31–57.

Kater, M. H. (1989) *Doctors Under Hitler* (University of North Carolina Press, Chapel Hill, NC).

Kaupen-Hass, H. (1986) *Der Griff Nach Der Bevölkerung* (Franz Greno, Nördlingen).

Kevles, D. J. (1985) *In the Name of Eugenics* (Alfred A. Knopf, New York).

Klee, E. (1983) *"Euthanasie" im NS-Staat: Die Vernichtung lebensunwerten Lebens* (S. Fischer Verlag, Frankfurt).

Kottow, M. H. (1988) Euthanasia after the Holocaust—Is it possible?: A report from the Federal Republic of Germany. *Bioethics* **2(1)**, 58–69.

Kreutzberg, G. W. (1990) Irrewege und Abgrunde von Wissenschaft. *Münchener Med. Wochenschr.* **132,26,** 16–19.

Krugman, S. (1986) The Willowbrook hepatitis studies revisited: Ethical aspects. *Rev. Infect. Dis.* **8(1),** 157–162.

Kudlien, F. (1985) *Aertze im Nationalsozialismus* (Kiepenheuer & Witsch, Cologne).

Lacquer, W. (1981) *Suppression of the Truth about Hitler's Final Solution* (Little Brown, Boston).

LaFont, M. (1987) *L'Extermination douce: La Mort de 40,000 Malades Mentaux dans les Hôpitaux Psychiatriques en France, sous le Régime de Vichy* (Editions de L'Arefppi, Paris).

Lasagna, L. (1977) Prisoners, subjects and drug testing. *Fed. Proc.* **36(10),** 2349–2351.

Lekisch, K. and McDonald, J. H. (1989) The politics of choice: Roles of the medical profession under Nazi rule. *Texas Med.* **85,** 32–39.

Lerner, R. M. (1992) *Final Solutions: Biology, Prejudice and Genocide* (Pennsylvania State University Press, University Park, PA).

Levine, R. J. (1981) *Ethics and Regulation of Clinical Research,* 2nd ed. (Urband and Schwarzenberg, Baltimore, MD).

Levine, C. (1989) Military medical research: 1. Are there ethical exceptions? *IRB* **11(4),** pp. 5–7.

Lifton, R. J. (1982) Medicalized killing in Auschwitz. *Psychiatry* **45(4)** 283–297.

Lifton, R. J. (1986) *The Nazi Doctors—Medical Killing and the Psychology of Genocide* (Basic Books, New York).

Maier, C. (1989) *The Unmasterable Past: History, Holocaust and German National Identity* (Harvard University Press, Cambridge, MA).

Maretzki, T. W. (1989) The documentation of Nazi medicine by German medical sociologists: A review. *Soc. Sci. Med.* **29(12),** 1319–1322.

Martin, R. M. (1986) Using Nazi scientific data. *Dialogue (Canada)* **25**, 403–411.

Mayer, A. J. (1989) *Why Did the Heavens Not Darken? The "Final Solution" in History* (Pantheon, New York).

Mellanby, K. (1973) *Human Guinea Pigs* (Merlin Press, London).

Mellanby, K. (1975) Experiments on human volunteers. *J. Biosociol. Sci.* **7**, 189–195.

Meyer, J. E. (1988) 'Die Freigabe der Vernichtung lebensunwerten Lebens' von Binding und Hoche im Spiegel der deutschen Psychiatrie vor 1933. ('The release for extermination of those unworthy of living' by Binding and Hoche: the response of German psychiatry prior to 1933.) *Nervenarzt* **59**, 85–91.

Meyer, J. E. (1988) The fate of the mentally ill in Germany during the Third Reich. *Psychol. Med.* **18**, 575–581.

Meyer, E. (1989) Nazi-period cadavers still used in West and East German universities. *Jerusalem Post* **6**, p. 2.

Miles, S. H. (1989) Review of: Race hygiene and national efficiency: The eugenics of Wilhelm Schallmayer. *JAMA* **261(2)**, 300,301.

Mitscherlich, A. and Mielke, F. (1949) *Doctors of Infamy*. Henry Schuman, New York.

Moe, K. (1984) Should the Nazi research data be cited? *Hastings Cent. Rep.* **14**, p. 7.

Moss, R. (1987) The abuse of medicine as a political power in Nazi Germany. *Med. War* **3(1)**, 43–48.

Musqat, M. (1985) The Mengele file. *Int. Probl.* **24(1–4)**, 25–31.

Müller-Hill, B. (1987) Genetics after Auschwitz. *Holocaust Genocide Stud.* **2(1)**, 3–20.

Müller-Hill, B. (1988) From eugenics to genocide. *Nature* **334**, 573,574.

Müller-Hill, B. (1988) *Murderous Science. Elimination by Scientific Selection of Jews, Gypsies and Others, Germany 1933–1945* (trans. G. Fraser), Oxford University Press, Oxford, UK.

Neuhaus, R. J. (1988) The return of eugenics. *Commentary* **85**, pp. 15–26.

Nixon, A. (1988) If the data's good, use it—regardless of the source. *The Scientist* **14**, 9,11.

Noakes, J. and Pridham, G., eds. (1988) The 'Euthanasia' Programme 1939–1945. *Exeter Studies in History 13* (Exeter University Publications), 997–1048.

Nyiszli, M. (1960) *Auschwitz* (Fawcett, New York).

Orlans, F. B. (1985) Nazi research: Too evil to cite. (Letter to Ed.) *Hastings Cent. Rep.* **15**, 31,32.

Pappworth, M. H. (1968) *Human Guinea Pigs: Experimentation On Man* (Beacon Press, Boston).

Peiffer, J. (1991) Neuropathology in the Third Reich: Memorial to those victims of the National–Socialist atrocities in Germany who were used by medical science. *Brain Pathol.* **1**, 125–131.

Pence, G. E. (1988) Do not go slowly into that dark night: Mercy killing in Holland. *Am. J. Med.* **84**, 139–141.

Pfäfflin, F. (1986) The connection between eugenics, sterilization and mass murder in Germany from 1933 to 1945. *Med. Law* **5**, 11–15.

Pittsburgh Press (1988, Aug. 11) Report details Japan's wartime experiments on prisoners. p. A4.

Pois, R. A. (1988) Uses of biology. *Science* **242**, 785–787.

Post, S. G. (1989) Nazi data and the rights of Jews. *J. Law Religion* **6(2)**, 101–105.

Powell, J. (1981) Japan's biological weapons 1930–1945. A hidden chapter in history. *Bull. Atomic Sci.* **37(3)**, 44–53.

Proctor, R. N. (1988) *Racial Hygiene: Medicine under the Nazis* (Harvard University Press, Cambridge, MA).

Proctor, R. N. (1988) Science and Nazism. *Science,* **241**, 730,731.

Proctor, R. N. (1990) Nazi health and social policy. *Simon Wiesenthal Annual* **7**, 145–167.

Pross, C. (1991) Breaking through the postwar coverup of Nazi doctors in Germany. *J. Med. Ethics* **17**, 13–16.

Rabinbach, A. (1988) German historians debate the Nazi past. *Dissent* **34**, 192–200.

Ramsey, P. (1970) *The Patient as Person* (Yale University Press, New Haven, CT).

Reilly, P. (1991) *The Surgical Solution* (Johns Hopkins University Press, Baltimore, MD).

Reiser, S. J. (1978) Human experimentation and the convergence of medical research and patient care. *Ann. Am. Acad. Pol. Soc. Sci.* **437**, pp. 64–70.

Remains of Nazi Victims Used by Universities. (1989) *The Globe and Mail (Canada)*, p. A11.

Roland, C. G. (1989) An underground medical school in the Warsaw ghetto, 1941–2. *Med. Hist.* **33**, 399–419.

Roscher, H. (1946) Medicine in Dachau. *Br. Med. J.* 953–955.

Rothman, D. J. Ethics of human experimentation: Henry Beecher revisited. *N. Engl. J. Med.* **317(19)**, 1195–119.

Rothman, D. J. (1982) Were Tuskegee and Willowbrook 'studies in nature'? *Hastings Cent. Rep.* **12**, 5–7.

Sass, H-M. (1983) Reichsrundschreiben 1931: Pre-Nuremberg German regulation concerning new therapy and human experimentation. *J. Med. Philos.* **8(2)**, 99–111.

Schafer, A. (1986) On using Nazi data: The case against. *Dialogue (Canada)* **25,** 413–419.

Schmuhl, H.-W. (1987) *Rassenhygiene, Nationalsozialismus, Euthanasie* (Vandenhoeck & Ruprecht, Göttingen).

Segal, N. L. (1985) Holocaust twins: Their special bond. *Psychol. Today* **19,** pp. 52–58.

Segal, N. L. (1985) Twin survivors of the Holocaust. *Twins* 28–31.

Segal, N. L. (1989) Twin survivors of Auschwitz-Birkenau: Behavioral, medical and social issues, in *Remembering for the Future* (Pergamon, Oxford, UK), pp. 2288–2298.

Seidelman, W. E. (1986) Animal experiments in Nazi Germany. *Lancet* p. 1214.

Seidelman, W. E. (1988) Mengele medicus: Medicine's Nazi heritage. *Milbank Q.* **66,** 221–239.

Seidelman, W. E. (1989) In Memoriam: Medicine's confrontation with evil. *Hastings Cent. Rep.* **19(6),** 5–6.

Seidelman, W. E. (1989) Legacy of the Nazis. *Nature* **341,** 180.

Seidelman, W. E. (1989) Medical selection: Auschwitz antecedents and effluent. *Holocaust Genocide Stud.* **4(4),** 435–448.

Shabecoff, P. (1988, Mar. 23) EPA bars use of data from Nazi experiments. *St. Petersburg Times,* p. 4a.

Shabecoff, P. (1988, Mar. 23) Head of EPA bars Nazi data in study on gas. *New York Times,* 1,17.

Shirer, W. L. (1960) *The Rise and Fall of the Third Reich* (Fawcett, Greenwich, CT).

Siegel, B. (1988, Oct. 30) Nazi data: A dilemma for science. *Los Angeles Times* 1, 12.

Singer, P. (1990) Bioethics and academic freedom. *Bioethics* **4(1),** 33–44.

Spicker, S., Alon, I., and De Vries, A., eds. (1988) *The Use of Human Beings in Research* (Kluwer, Dordrecht).

Spiro, H. M. (1984) Eppinger of Vienna: Scientist and villain? *J. Clin. Gastroenterol.* **6,** 493–497.

Spiro, H. M. (1985) Nazi research: Too evil to cite. (Letter to Ed.) *Hastings Cent. Rep.* **15,** 31,32.

Spiro, H. M. (1988, Apr. 19) Let Nazi medical data remind us of evil. (Letter to Ed.) *New York Times,* p. 37.

Stein, G. J. (1988) Biological science and the roots of Nazism. *Am. Sci.* **76,** 50–58.

Steinsaltz, A. (1980) *The Thirteen Petalled Rose* (Basic Books, New York).

Sun, M. (1988) EPA bars use of Nazi data. *Science* **240,** p. 21.

Sykes, C. J. (1987) *Medical Nightmares: German Doctors/American Doctors* (Catholic League for Religious and Civil Rights).

(1988, Mar. 25) EPA bars use of Nazi data. *US News and World Report* p. 204.

(1988, Apr. 4) Good from evil?, *Time* 131, 68(1).

(1988, May 12) Minnesota scientist plans to publish a Nazi study; are death camp experiments a fit subject of scientific inquiry? *New York Times,* p. A28.

(1985, Feb. 18) Visions of Hell; pursuing the 'Angel of Death' *Time* 125, p. 54.

(1948) *Trials of War Criminals Before the Nuremberg Military Tribunals; The Medical Case,* vols. 1,2, (US Government Printing Office, Washington, DC).

Tyrnauer, G. (1984) Action and ethics in applied anthropology. *Kölner Zeitschrift für Soziologie und Sozialpsychologie,* Suppl. 26, 113–123.

Wallis, C. (1984) Infamy haunts a top award; A research prize is canceled because of a Nazi connection. *Time* 124, p. 89.

Walsh, M. (1989) Nazi research under the microscope. *Time* 133(9), pp. 53,54.

Ward, M. P., Milledgo, J. S., and West, J. B. (1989) *High Altitude Medicine and Physiology* (University of Pennsylvania, Philadelphia).

Weingart, P. (1987) The rationalization of sexual behavior: The institutionalization of eugenic thought in Germany. *J. Hist. Biol.* 20(2), pp. 159–193.

Weingart, P., Kroll, J., and Bayertz, K., eds. (1988) *Rasse, Blut und Gene: Geschichte der Eugenik und Rassenhygiene in Deutschland* (Suhrkamp Verlag, Frankfurt am Main).

Weindling, P. (1985) Weimar eugenics: The Kaiser Wilhelm Institute for Anthropology, Human Heredity and Eugenics in social context. *Ann. Sci.* 42, 303–318.

Weindling, P. (1988) The Rockefeller Foundation and German Biomedical Sciences, 1920–40, in *Science, Politics and the Public* (Rupke, N. A., ed.), Macmillan, London, 119–140.

Weinreich, M. (1946) *Hitler's Professors* (Yiddish Scientific Institute, New York).

Weiskopf, M. (1988) EPA bars use of Nazis' human test data after scientists object. *Washington Post* 111, p. a17.

Weiss, S. F. (1987) *Race Hygiene and National Efficiency: The Eugenics of Wilhelm Schallmayer* (University of California Press, Berkeley, CA).

Wertham, F. (1980) The geranium in the window: The 'euthanasia' murders, in *Death, Dying and Euthanasia* (Horan, D. J., ed.), University Publications of America, Washington, DC.

Whymant, R. (1983) The butchers of Harbin: experiments on POWs—
Japan World War II. *Conn. Med.* **47,3,** 163–165.

Williams, P. and Wallace, D. (1989) *Unit 731* (Hodder & Stoughton,
London).

Winick, M. (1979) *Hunger Disease: Studies by the Jewish physicians
in the Warsaw Ghetto* (Wiley, New York).

Zofka, Z. (1986) The concentration camp doctor, Josef Mengele: Typology
of a Nazi criminal. *Vierteljahrshefte für Zeitgeschichte* **34(2),**
245–267.

Notes and References

Konopka Chapter

[1]Anderson, M. (1949) *Joan of Lorraine,* Menasha, WI, p. 91
[2]Solzhenitsyn, A. *The First Circle*, p. 343.

Proctor Chapter

[1]A similar version of this paper appears in Casey, T. and Embree, L., eds. (1989) *Lifeworld and Technology* (University Press, Washington, DC). For a more elaborate account of the argument presented here, *see* Proctor, R. N. (1988) *Racial Hygiene: Medicine Under the Nazis* (Harvard University Press, Cambridge, MA).
[2]The *Encyclopedia of Philosophy* (1967) suggests that unlike Marxism, fascism and Nazism "were not coherent doctrines, and their proponents never made more than a pretense of reconciling theory and practice" (vol. 6, p. 385). Another article states that National Socialism "had no doctrine in the proper sense of the word. It was fundamentally hostile to philosophy, and the ideas of orthodoxy and heresy remained foreign to it...The ideas—few in number, and crude as well as shallow—that formed the hard core of the national socialist creed had hardly sufficient logical coherence to deserve the name of ideology...National Socialism was a perversion of philosophy rather than a philosophy" (vol. 3, pp. 309,310).
[3]I use the term *flourish* in a qualified and deliberately provocative sense. It is important to distinguish not only between different sciences in this regard (e.g., between human genetics and theoretical physics), but also between different senses of the term "flourish." I am not claiming that *all* sciences flourished, nor that science flourished in a moral or theoretical sense. I mean that science (only certain sciences, and only for a time) flourished in a professional or purely *quantitative* sense—numbers of journal articles published, research expenditures, and so on. One cannot doubt that science

331

as a whole suffered profoundly in both a moral and theoretical sense during this period. Morally, science is put in the service of oppressive injustice and ultimately genocide; theoretically, the position of world leadership occupied by German science prior to 1933 was largely destroyed by the expulsion of the Jews and the reign of terror imposed by Nazi rule. The collapse of Germany during the war dealt a further blow to German scientific institutions from which modern Germany has not fully recovered.

[4]Interestingly, those areas of science that were suppressed by the Nazis—relativity theory, for example, or quantum mechanics—have been those that have, until recently, received the most attention from historians and sociologists. This is probably owing to the fact that these fit the traditional image of the fate of science under totalitarian rule—namely, that scientific progress and totalitarian rule are mutually incompatible.

[5]Siemens, H. W. (1916/1918) Was ist Rassenhygiene? *Archiv für Rassen- und Gesellschaftsbiologie* **12**, 281,282.

[6]Ploetz, A. (1895) *Die Tüchtigkeit unsrer Rasse und der Schutz der Schwachen* (Fischer Verlag, Berlin).

[7]Biologism (or biological determinism) is the view that "nature" is far more important than "nurture" in the formation of human character and institutions. Typically, it is the view that men and women, or different races, have different inborn talents or disabilities—that certain individuals, for example, are "born criminals," or that the occupations people choose are largely determined by their inherited capacities. *See* Lewontin, R., Rose, S., and Kamin, L. (1984) *Not In Our Genes* (Pantheon, New York).

[8]Lenz, F. (1931) *Menschliche Auslese und Rassenhygiene (Eugenik)*, 3rd ed. (J. F. Lehmann Verlag, Munich), p. 417.

[9]The fact that Americans had pioneered forcible sterilization was important in postwar deliberations concerning which among the Nazi racial programs should be considered war crimes. Nuremberg authorities generally did not consider forcible sterilization criminal. After the war, individuals who had been sterilized received compensation as victims of Nazi oppression only if they could prove they had been sterilized illegally—that is, only if they could prove they were not in fact genetically feeble-minded, alcoholic, epileptic, and so forth. The reason for this was obvious—that similar programs had been widespread in the US.

[10]Similar awards were not uncommon in other countries at this time. In 1926, a Toronto millionaire willed $700,000 to the Canadian woman who, by the year 1936, would have the most children. I do

not know who won, but as of 1930 there was a certain Mrs. Brown who, at the age of 40, had already given birth to 26 children!

[11]The May 15, 1939 census showed there were 380,892 Jews in the *Altreich* (Germany prior to the annexation of Austria), down from 722,000 in 1933. The census showed a ratio of women to men of 1,366 to 1,000. *See the Archiv für Rassen- und Gesellschaftsbiologie* **34** (1940–1941): 313.

[12]Bock, G. (1986) *Zwangssterilisation im Nationalsozialismus* (Westdeutscher Verlag, Opladen), p. 13.

[13]*See* Proctor, R. N. (1988) *Racial Hygiene: Medicine Under the Nazis* (Harvard University Press, Cambridge, MA), especially chapter 6.

[14]Keine Negerärzte in der amerikanischen Standesorganisation, *Archiv für Rassen- und Gesellschaftsbiologie* **33** (1939–1940): 276; also 33 (1939–1940): 96. In 1930 there were about 5000 black American physicians among a population of some 13,000,000 blacks. The appeal by America's black physicians was placed at the annual meeting of the AMA in St. Louis; the appeal was rejected. America's leading medical organization remained essentially a segregated body until the mid-1950s.

[15]Kennedy, F. (1942) The problem of social control of the congenitally defective: education, sterilization, euthanasia. *Am. J. Psychiatry* **99**, 13–16.

[16]Institut für Zeitgeschichte (1988) *Medizin im Nationalsozialismus* (Oldenbourg Verlag, Munich), pp. 24,25.

[17]*Ibid.*, pp. 25,26.

[18]After the war, the Nazi chief of police for occupied Warsaw (Arpad Wigand) defended shooting several thousand Jews attempting to leave the ghetto on the grounds that the area had been quarantined.

[19]Müller-Hill, B. (1988) *Murderous Science: Elimination by Scientific Selection of Jews, Gypsies, and Others, Germany 1933–1945* (Fraser, G. R., trans), Oxford University Press, Oxford, UK, p. 18.

[20]For the case of anthropology, *see* Proctor, R., ed. (1988) From *Anthropologie* to *Rassenkunde:* Concepts of race in German physical anthropology, in *Bones, Bodies, Behavior: Essays on Biological Anthropology*, Stocking, G. (University of Wisconsin Press, Madison).

[21]Many of the journals closed by the Nazi regime were associated with either communist or socialist causes. Journals primarily devoted to the economic affairs of the profession were also reorganized and began publishing once again only after the *Gleichschaltung* of the profession.

[22]One of the earliest uses of the term "sociobiology" in English can be found in the Nazi criminologist Hans von Hentig's book, translated into English in 1948. *The Criminal and his Victim, Studies in the Sociobiology of Crime* (Yale University Press, New Haven).
[23]In 1939, the city of Dresden enacted a law prohibiting smoking in all public buildings. *See Archiv für Rassen- und Gesellschaftsbiologie* **33** (1939–1940): 274.
[24]Wertham, F. (1966) *A Sign for Cain* (Macmillan, New York), p. 167.

Müller-Hill Chapter

[1]Nochmals, L. K. (1940) Systematik und Entwicklungsgedanke im Unterricht. *Der Biologe* **9**, 24–36.
[2]Müller-Hill, B. (1988) *Murderous Science. Elimination by Scientific Selection of Jews, Gypsies and Others, Germany 1933–1945* (Fraser, G. R., trans.), Oxford University Press, Oxford, UK.
[3]Proctor, R. N. (1988) *Racial Hygiene: Medicine under the Nazis* (Harvard University Press, Cambridge, MA).
[4]Munchow, R. (1943) 950 Gutachten in Erbgesundheitssachen der Jahre 1934–1940. Ph.D. Dissertation, Berlin University.
[5]Wilkerson, I. (1989, May 21) Nazi scientists and ethics of today. *The New York Times*, p. 34.
[6]Kater, M. H. (1974) *Das "Ahnenerbe" der SS 1933–1945. Ein Beitrag zur Kulturpolitik des Dritten Reiches* (Deutsche Verlagsanstalt, Stuttgart).
[7]Benz, W. (1988) Dr. med. Sigmund Rascher. *Dachauer Hefte* **4**, 190–214.
[8]Kant, I. (1977) Über ein vermeintes Recht aus Menschenliebe zu lugen. *Berlinische Blätter* 1797; **1**, 301-304, reprint in *Werkausgabe* (Suhrkamp Verlag Frankfurt) **8**, 637–643.

Caplan Chapter

[1]Annas, G., ed. (1992) *The Nuremberg Code* (Oxford Univ. Press, New York).
[2]Lifton, R. J. (1986) *The Nazi Doctors* (Basic Books, New York).
[3]Berger, R.L. (1990) Nazi science—The Dachau hypothermia experiments. *N. Engl. J. Med.* **322(20)**, 1435–1440.
[4]Seidelman, W. E. (1988) Mengele medicus: Medicine's nazi heritage. *Milbank Q.* **66**, 221-239.
[5]Proctor, R. N. (1988) *Racial Hygiene: Medicine Under the Nazis* (Harvard University Press, Cambridge, MA).
[6]Kater, M. H. (1989) *Doctors Under Hitler* (University of North Carolina Press, Chapel Hill, NC).
[7]Müller-Hill, B. (1987) Genetics after Auschwitz. *Holocaust Genocide Stud.* **2(1)**, 3–20.

[8]Shannon, T. A., ed. (1976) *Bioethics* (Paulist Press, New York).

[9]Munson, R., ed. (1983) *Intention and Reflection: Basic Issues in Medical Ethics*, 2nd. ed. (Wadsworth, Belmont, CA).

[10]Beauchamp, T. and Walters, L., eds. (1982) *Contemporary Issues in Bioethics,* 2nd. ed. (Wadsworth, Belmont, CA).

[11]Mappes, T. A. and Zembaty, J. S. (1991) *Biomedical Ethics* (McGraw-Hill, New York).

[12]Rothman, D. (1991) *Strangers at the Bedside* (Basic, NY, NY).

[13]Caplan, A. L. (1990) Telling it like it wasn't, *Hastings Cent. Rep.* **March/April,** 47,48.

[14]Müller-Hill, B. (1988) *Murderous Science: Elimination by Scientific Selection of Jews, Gypsies and Others, Germany 1933–1945* (Fraser, G., trans.), Oxford University Press, Oxford, UK.

[15]Vawter, D., Keamey, W., Gervais, K., Caplan, A. L., Garry, D., and Tauer, C. (1990) *The Use of Human Fetal Tissue: Scientific, Ethical and Policy Concerns* (Center for Biomedical Ethics, Minneapolis, MN).

[16]Burtchaell, J. and Bopp, J. (1988) Statement of Dissent, Human Fetal Tissue Transplantation Panel (National Institutes of Health, Bethesda, MD), pp. 1–31.

[17]Caplan, A. L. (1990) The end of a myth. *Dimensions: J. Holocaust Stud.* **5,2,** 13–18.

[18]Moe, K. (1984) Should the nazi research data be cited? *Hastings Cent. Rep.* **14,** 5–7.

[19](1948)*Trials of War Criminals Before the Nuremberg Military Tribunals; The Medical Case,* vols. 1,2 (US Government Printing Office, Washington, DC).

[20]British Broadcasting Corporation (1990) "Nazi Science, Antennae."

[21](Sources: Nuremberg Trial transcripts; transcripts of various war crimes trials, Proctor, *Racial Hygiene; IME Bulletin,* Feb. 1989; Müller-Hill, *Murderous Science;* J. E. Meyer, "The fate of the mentally ill in Germany during the Third Reich", 1988; R. Proctor, personal communications, 1989).

Pozos Chapter

[1]Jonsen, A. R. and Toulmin, S. (1988) *The Abuse of Casuistry—A History of Moral Reasoning* (University of California Press, Los Angeles, CA), pp. 65–68, 342, 343.

[2]Alexander, L. (1949) Medical science under dictatorship. *N. Engl. J. Med.* **241,2,** 39–47.

[3]Katz, J. (1979) *Experimentation with Human Beings* (Russell Sage Foundation, New York), pp. 733,734.

[4]Caplan, A. and Pozos, R. (1988) Personal communication.

[5]Lifton, R. (1986) *The Nazi Doctors: Medical Killing and the Psychology of Genocide* (Basic Books, New York).

[6]Proctor, R. N. (1988) *Racial Hygiene: Medicine Under the Nazis* (Harvard University Press, Cambridge, MA).

[7](1946)*Trials of War Criminals Before the Nuremberg Military Tribunal,* part 3 (His Majesty's Stationery Office, London).

[8](1949)*Trials of War Criminals Before the Nuremberg Military Tribunals Under Control Council Law No. 10.* vol 1, 197–278.

[9]Analysis of the scientific literature from 1930–1940 revealed no papers concerning the topic of Human Response to Immersion Hypothermia.

[10]Golden, FStC. (1979) Physiological Changes in Immersion Hypothermia with Special Reference to Factors Which may Be Responsible for Death in the Early Rewarming Phase. Ph.D. Thesis, University of Leeds.

[11]Berben, P. (1968) *Dachau. The Official History 1933–1945* (Norfolk Press, London).

[12]Alexander, L. (1946) *The Treatment of Shock from Prolonged Exposure to Cold Especially in Water.* Item No. 24, #250 (Office of Publication Board, Dept. of Commerce, Washington, DC).

[13]*Ibid.*, part 22.

[14]*Ibid.*, part 21.

[15]*Ibid.,* part 8.

[16]Mitscherlich, A. and Mielke, F. (1949) *Doctors of Infamy, The Story of the Nazi Medical Crimes* (Henry Schuman, New York).

[17]Golden, FStC. (1988) *Accidental Hypothermia and Near Drowning* (Gallandat Huet, R. C. G., Euverman, Th. S. M., Coad, N. R., de Vos, R., and Karliczek, G. I., eds.), Van Gorcum, Assen Maastricht.

[18]*Ibid.*, part 5.

[19]Beecher, H. K. (1966) *N. Engl. J. Med.* **274,** 1354–1360.

[20]*Ibid.,* part 4.

[21]Ivy, A. C. (1947) Nazi war crimes of a medical nature. *Fed. Bull.* **33,** 133–147.

[22]Nestor, J. and Pozos, R., personal communication.

[23]Adolph, E. F. and Molnar, G. W. (1946)*Am. J. Physiol.* **146,** 507–537.

[24]Burton, A. C. and Otto G. E. (1969) *Man in a Cold Environment: Physiological and Pathological Effects of Exposure to Low Temperatures* (Hafner Publishing, New York).

[25]Covino, B. G. (1958) *Cold Injury* (Irene, M., ed.), Ferrar, New York.

[26]Felix, R., Rosenhain, K. E., and Penrod, K. E. (1951)*Am. J. Physiol.* **166,** 55–61.

[27]Harrington, L. P. (1968) *Physiology of Heat Regulation and the Science of Clothing* (Newburgh, L. H., ed.), Hafner Publishing, New York, pp. 262–275.

[28]Molar, A. C. (1946) *JAMA* **131**, 1046.

[29]Steinman, A. M. and Hayward, J. S. (1989) *Management and Wilderness and Environmental Emergencies* (Auerbach, P. S. and Geehr, E. C., eds.), Mosby, St. Louis, MO.

[30]Wayburn, E. (1947) *Arch. Intern. Med.* **79**, 77–91.

[31]Bigelow, W. G., Lindsay, W. K., and Greenwood, W. F. (1950) *Ann. Surg.* **132**, 849–866.

[32]Hegnauer, A. H., Flynn, J., and D'Amato, H. (1951) *Am. J. Physiol.* **167**, 69–71.

[33]Hegnauer, A. H. (1959) *Ann. NY Acad. Sci.* **80**, 315–319.

[34]Nestor, J. (1955) *Med. Ann. DC.* **XXIV**, 239–241.

[35]Lange, K., Weiner, D., and Gold, M. (1949) *Ann. Intern. Med.* **31**, 989–1002.

[36]Beecher, H. K. (1965) *Experimentation in Man* (Charles C. Thomas, Springfield, IL).

[37]Moe, K. (1984) Should the Nazi research data be cited? *Hastings Cent. Rep.* pp. 5–7.

Berger Chapter

[1](1946–1949)*Trials of War Criminals Before Nuremberg Military Tribunals. The Medical Case*, vol. 1 (US Government Printing Office, Washington, DC), 28.

[2]Affidavit by Blaha, F. (1948) *Trials of War Criminals Before the Nuremberg Military Tribunals,* vol. 5. (Secretariat of the Tribunal, Nuremberg, Germany) 168–172.

[3]Mitscherlich, A. and Mielke, F. (1949) *Doctors of Infamy* (Henry Schuman, New York).

[4]Alexander, L. (1946) *The Treatment of Shock from Prolonged Exposure to Cold, Especially in Water.* (US Department of Commerce, Washington, DC).

[5]Freezing experiments (1946–1949) *Trials of War Criminals Before the Nuremberg Military Tribunals,* vol. 1 (US Government Printing Office, Washington, DC), 198–217.

[6]Alexander, L. (1949) Medical science under dictatorship. *N. Engl. J. Med.* **241**, 39–47.

[7]Pozos, R. (1989) Can scientists use information derived from concentration camps? Conference on the Meaning of the Holocaust for Bioethics. University of Minnesota, Minneapolis, MN. Transcription of official recording.

[8]Moe, K. (1984) Should the Nazi research data be cited? *Hastings Cent. Rep.* pp. 5–7.

[9]Gagge, A. P. and Harrington, L. P. (1947) Physiological effects of heat and cold. *Ann. Rev. Physiol.* **9**, 409–427.

[10]Laufman, H. (1951) Profound accidental hypothermia. *JAMA* **147**, 1201–1212.

[11]Berger, R. L. (1990) Nazi science—The Dachau human hypothermia experiments. *N. Engl. J. Med.* **322**, 1435–1440.

[12]Letter from Rascher, S. to Brandt, R. (1946–1949) *Trials of War Criminals Before the Nuremberg Military Tribunals,* vol. 1. (US Government Printing Office, Washington, DC), 221,222.

[13]Benz, W. (1988) Dr med Sigmund Rascher Eine Karriere. Medizin in NS-Staat. *Dachauer Hefte.* **4 (4)**, 190–214.

[14]Angell, M. (1990) The Nazi hypothermia experiments and unethical research today. *N. Engl. J. Med.* **322**, 1462–1464.

[15]Rosner, F., Bennett, A. J., Cassell, E. J., et al. (1991) The ethics of using scientific data obtained by immoral means. *NY State J. Med.* **91**, 54–59.

[16]Lutz, D. (1990, May 17) Surgeon calls Nazi hypothermia research bad science. *The Minnesota Daily,* 12.

[17]Katz, J. and Pozos, R. S. (1991) The Dachau hypothermia study— an ethical and scientific commentary. Personal communication. Paper submitted for publication.

[18]Golden, FStC. (1991) Nazi Science. Antenna Program. British Broadcasting Corporation.

[19]Wilkerson, I. (1989, May 21) Nazi scientists and ethics of today. *New York Times,* p. 34.

[20]Siegel, B. (1988, Oct. 30) Nazi data: A dilemma for science. *Los Angeles Times.*

[21]Mills, D. (1988) Use of Nazi data an ethical morass. *Insight* 50,51.

[22]Public Broadcast System (1988, Aug. 1) *McNeil-Lehrer Report.*

[23]Columbia Broadcast System (1988, June 19) *Newswatch.*

[24]WNEV-TV (1990, Jan. 20) *Our Times.*

[25]Caplan, A. (1988, April 25) Data too tainted with horror to be of use? *St. Paul Pioneer Dispatch,* 1B.

[26]Rascher, S. Intermediate report (1946–1949) *Trials of War Criminals Before the Nuremberg Military Tribunals,* vol. 1 (US Government Printing Office, Washington, DC), 220,221.

[27]Froese, G. and Burton, A. C. (1957) Heat losses from the human head. *J. Appl. Physiol.* **10**, 235–241.

[28]Hayward, J. S., Collis, M., and Eckinson, J. D. (1973) Thermographic evaluation of relative heat loss of man during cold water immersion. *Aerospace Med.* **44**, 708–711.

[29]Testimony of Pacholegg, A. (1947) *Nazi conspiracy and aggression*. International Military Tribunal. Suppl A. (US Government Printing Office, Washington, DC), 414–422.

[30]Danzl, D. F., Pozos, R. F., and Hamlet, M. P. (1989) Accidental hypothermia, in *Management of Wilderness and Environmental Emergencies*. Auerbach, P. S. and Geehr, E. J., eds., Mosby, St. Louis, MO.

[31]Grosse-Bruckhoff, F. Discussion of Paper by Holzloehner. Doc No. 401, in *The Alexander Papers. Special Collections*. Mugar Memorial Library, Boston University, Boston, MA.

[32]Grosse-Bruckhoff, F. (1946) Pathologic physiology and therapy of hypothermia, in *German Aviation Medicine During WW II* (Department of Air Force. Surgeon General, Washington, DC), pp. 828–842.

[33]Lifton, R. L. (1986) *Nazi Doctors* (Basic Books, New York).

[34]Testimony of Neff, W. (1946–1949) *Trials of War Criminals Before the Nuremberg Military Tribunals*, vol. 1 (US Government Printing Office, Washington, DC), 260–265.

[36]Deposition of Neff, W. (1946) *The Alexander Papers. Special Collections*. Mugar Memorial Library, Boston University, Boston, MA.

[35]Berben, P. (1975) *Dachau 1933–1945: The Official History* (Norfolk Press, London).

[37]*Directory of Medical Specialists*. vol 2. Chicago, IL. Marquis Who's Who, 1972–1973, 1486.

[38]Bigelow, W. G., Callaghan, J. C., and Hopps, J. A. (1950) General hypothermia for experimental intracardiac surgery. *Ann. Surg.* **132**, 531–539.

[39]Lewis, F. J. and Taufic, M. (1953) Closure of atrial septal defects with the aid of hypopthermia; experimental accomplishments and report of one successful case. *Surgery* **33**, 52–59.

[40]Zeavin, I., Virtue, R. W., and Swan, H. (1954) Cessation of circulation in general hypothermia. II Anesthetic management. *Anesthesiology* **15**, 113–121.

[41]Nestor, J. O., Walsh, B. J., Davis, E. W., and Fierst, C. E. (1955) The use of hypothermia in cardiac surgery, including a report of four patients. *Med. Ann. Dist. Col.* **24**, 107–111.

[42]*Ibid.*, *Clin. Proc. Children's Hosp.* Washington DC, 1955, **11**, 108–114.

[43]Talbot, J. H., Consolazio, W. V., and Pecora, L. J. (1941) Hypothermia. Report of a case in which the patient died during therapeutic reduction of body temperature, with metabolic and pathologic studies. *Arch. Int. Med.* **68**, 1120–1132.

[44]Fay, T. (1959) Early experiences with local and generalized refrigeration of the human brain. *J. Neurosurg.* **16**, 239–260.

[45]Sealy, W. C. (1989) Hypothermia: Its possible role in cardiac surgery. *Ann. Thor. Surg.* **47**, 788–791.

[46]Nazi data: Dissociation from evil. *Hastings Cent. Rep.* July/August, 16–18.

[47]Caplan, A. (1989) Examining the ethics of the unspeakable: The holocaust and biomedical ethics. Conference on The Meaning of the Holocaust for Bioethics. University of Minnesota, Minneapolis, MN.

Katz and Pozos Chapter

[1]Berger, R. L. (1990) Nazi science—The Dachau hypothermia experiments. *N. Engl. J. Med.* 1435–1440.

[2]*Ibid.*, p. 1437.

[3]*Ibid.*, p. 1436.

[4]*Ibid.*, p. 1436,1437.

[5]*Ibid.*, p. 1437.

[6]*Ibid.*, p. 1438.

[7]*Ibid.*, p. 1438 (emphasis supplied).

[8]Wade, N. (1990, May 27) The errors of nazi science. *The New York Times.*

[9]Angell, M. (1990) The nazi hypothermia experiments and unethical research today. *N. Engl. J. Med.* 1463.

[10]*Ibid.*

Freedman Chapter

[1]For an explanation of these concepts, *see* my Scientific value and validity as ethical requirements for research. *IRB: A Rev. Hum. Subjects Res.* **9**, pp. 7–10.

[2]The following discussion is confined to the moral question of the use of data. Among the associated but separate moral questions that arise is the proper disposition of human tissue specimens gathered in the course of the Nazi project, which remained on display at Tübingen for many years. This moral question poses no dilemma to my mind. There is only one humanly decent response to the question of the specimens: solemn burial.

[3]Berger, R. L. (1990) Nazi science—The Dachau human hypothermia experiments. *N. Engl. J. Med.* **322,** 1435–1440.

[4]Seidelman, W., this vol. Murder as 'medspeak': Euthanasia, medicalized killing, and medical experimentation in Nazi Germany, this vol.

[5]See statements of Gen. Telford Taylor and responses of the Nazi defendants, quoted in Katz, J., Capron, A., and Glass, E., eds. (1972)

Experimentation with Human Beings (Russell Sage Foundation, New York), pp. 295–305; from (1948) *Trials of War Criminals Before the Nuremberg Military Tribunals, The Medical Case,* vols. 1,2 (US Government Printing Office, Washington, DC).

[6]Barber, B., Lally, J. J., Makarushka, J. L., and Sullivan, D. (1973) *Research on Human Subjects: Problems of Social Control in Medical Experimentation* (Russell Sage Foundation, New York). *See* especially chapters 4 and 5.

[7]Levine, R. J. (1986) *Ethics and Regulation of Clinical Research,* 2nd ed. (Urban & Schwarzenberg, Baltimore, MD). *See* discussion at pp. 28–31.

[8]A discussion by Lord Immanuel Jakobovits, Chief Rabbi of Great Britain, came to my attention after initial preparation of this paper. He employs a version of this symbolic argument, and writes as follows:

"[W]hat troubles me personally is the implicit claim that some good might be derived from this evil...What is at stake here, I believe, is not just a matter of semantics, nor is it the condoning of Nazi crimes. It is the basic moral question [sic] whether any good of any significance resulted from the most evil mass perversity in human history. Even if it did, it would not make the evil any lesser. But if it did not, as I have always so far assumed on the basis of the medical evidence available to me, then at least we can claim that medicine did not gain from experiments carried out on a massive scale in violation of the most elementary human rights. A constant reminder of this fact, if it could be established beyond all doubt, might serve as a powerful warning to the present and future generations never again to sanction unethical methods for the dubious benefits of medical or scientific advances. If that lesson were to be learned from the Nazi prostitution of medicine, it would indeed be the one 'direct benefit to humanity' which no one could dispute." Lord Immanuel Jakobovits (1988) Some modern responses on medico-moral problems, *Jewish Med. Ethics* **1,** 5–16 at 9,10.

The statement is puzzling on several accounts. It is clearly a matter of contingent fact whether the results of the experiments were or are of use, rather than a matter of moral concern. (Rabbi Jakobovits indicates as much when he states in his discussion that if the experiments yielded therapeutic benefit "I would obviously have to revise assumptions I have made...") In Jakobovit's view, the experiments were unscientific as well as unethical, and therefore should seem to be *disqualified* from serving as a "warning... never again to sanction unethical methods" for an unethical practitioner *with genuine fealty to scientific method*. Jakobovits himself seeks a benefit—moral rather than scientific—by referring to the results, but to *achieve* that benefit he would require the research to be of valid therapeutic interest. He seems to be saying further that whereas the presence of valid data would not have diminished the wrong, the *absence* of useful data somehow adds gravity to the wrong—for we cannot then say after the *Shoa* that "at least" medicine *did* gain. These claims are not logically possible; but at any rate his statement may have meant something else. I find it, finally, puzzling that Rabbi Jakobovits in this responsum fails to refer to any Jewish source for purposes of analysis.

9Burtchaell, J. (1988) Case study: University policy on experimental use of aborted fetal tissue. *IRB Rev. Hum. Subjects Res.* **10,** 7–11.

10The attack upon the Israelites in the wilderness of Sinai by the nation of Amalek, described in *Exodus* xvii. 8–16, is understood by tradition as the archetype for all future persecution of the Jews, and is one of several events and injunctions whose daily recollection is incumbent upon each Jew.

11Freedman, B. (1989) "Ethics and Human Experiments: What Legacy From the Holocaust?" Presented for the Montreal Holocaust Centre, unpublished; draft available from the author.

12Rabbi Adin Steinsaltz (1980) *The Thirteen Petalled Rose* (Basic Books, New York), pp. 103,104.

13Proctor, R. N. (1988) *Racial Hygiene: Medicine Under the Nazis* (Harvard University Press, Cambridge, MA), p. 175.

14The following five paragraphs are taken from my unpublished paper, "Ethics and Human Experimentation: What Legacy From the Holocaust?" noted above.

15Lifton, R. J. (1986) *The Nazi Doctors: Medical Killing and the Psychology of Genocide* (Basic Books, New York), p. 108.

16*Ibid.*, pp. 31,32

17Drawn from Lifton's discussion, p. 72.

18I am grateful to Arthur Caplan for suggesting this point.

[19]For what it is worth, my own view is that emotion must supplement, but not supplant reason.

Greene Chapter

[1]The terminology is rather eclectic and can be confusing and even controversial. To simplify matters and facilitate understanding, the following "definitions" should help: *Torah*, the written and oral instruction transmitted by Moses; *Talmud*, the body of oral Torah that is the basis of Jewish law; *Repsonsa*, rabbinic rulings to specific legal questions; *Halakha,* the consensus ruling, "the path on which to walk."

Macklin Chapter

[1]Beauchamp, T. L. and Davidson, A. I. (1983) The definition of euthanasia, in *Moral Problems in Medicine,* 2nd ed. (Gorovitz. S., et al., eds.), Prentice-Hall, Englewood Cliffs, NJ, p. 453.

[2]Kronberg, M. H. (1988) in *How to Stop the Resurgence of Nazi Euthanasia Today,* Spannaus, N. B., Kronberg, M. H., and Everett, L., eds., *EIR Special Report* p. 129.

[3]*Ibid.,* pp. 130,131.

[4]Hentoff, N. (1988) Contested terrain: The nazi analogy in bioethics. *Hastings Cent. Rep.* **18,** p. 29.

[5]*Ibid.*

[6]Neuhaus, R. J. (1988) The return of eugenics. *Commentary* **July**, p. 15.

[7]*Ibid.*, p. 20.

[8]*Ibid.*, p. 15.

[9]"The Way They Were, the Way We Are," Richard John Neuhaus, this vol.

[10]*Ibid.*, ms. p. 26.

[11]Beauchamp and Davidson, p. 448.

[12]*Ibid.*, p. 456.

[13]*Ibid.*, p. 457.

[14]Cohen, C. B. (1983) 'Quality of life' and the analogy with the nazis. *J. Med. Philos.* **8,** p. 114. *See also* Cohen's commentary in Contested terrain: The nazi analogy in bioethics. *Hastings Cent. Rep.* **18,** pp. 32,33.

[15]Lorber, J. (1975) Ethical problems in the management of myelomeningocele and hydrocephalus. *J. Royal College of Physicians* **10,1**, 47–60.

[16]Dawidowicz, L. (1985) *Should the Baby Live?* (Kuhse, H. and Singer, P., eds.), Oxford University Press, New York, p. 94.

[17]Beauchamp and Davidson, p. 446, 447, 457.

[18]*Ibid.*, p. 446.

[19]*Ibid.*, p. 449.

[20]Noakes, J. and Pridham, G., eds. (1988) *Nazism 1919–1945, vol. 3, Foreign Policy, War and Racial Extermination*, Exeter Studies in History No. 13 (Exeter University Publications, Exeter, UK).

[21]*Ibid.*, p. 997.

[22]Beauchamp and Davidson, p. 453.

[23]*Ibid.*

[24]Proctor, R. N. (1988) *Racial Hygiene: Medicine Under the Nazis* (Harvard University Press, Cambridge, MA), p. 187.

[25]Noakes and Pridham, p. 1005; *See also* Lifton, R. J. (1986) *The Nazi Doctors* (Basic Books, New York), pp. 50,51.

[26]Noakes and Pridham, p. 1005 (statement of Karl Brandt from Nuremberg Trial).

[27]*Ibid.*, p. 1005.

[28]Kuhse and Singer, p. 12.

[29]*Ibid.*

[30]Noakes and Pridham, p. 1006.

[31]*Ibid.*, p. 1007.

[32]Lifton, R. J. (1986) *The Nazi Doctors: Medical Killing and the Psychology of Genocide* (Basic Books, New York), p. 54.

[33]Noakes and Pridham, p. 1007.

[34]Lifton, p. 55.

[35]Kuhse and Singer, p. 93.

[36]Kuhse and Singer, p. 95.

[37]Lamb, D. (1988) *Down the Slippery Slope: Arguing in Applied Ethics* (Croom Helm, New York), pp. 28,29.

[38]Crile, G. Jr. (1984, Dec. 19) The right to life. *Medical Tribune*, p. 27.

[39]Proctor, p. 182.

[40]Noakes and Pridham, p. 1010.

[41]Proctor, p. 191.

[42]Lifton, p. 65.

[43]*Ibid.*, p. 96.

[44]Noakes and Pridham, pp. 1010,1011.

[45]*Ibid*, p. 1017.

[46]*Ibid.*, p. 1013.

[47]*Ibid.*, p. 1018.

[48]*Ibid.*, p. 1043.

[49]Neuhaus, p. 24.

[50]*Ibid.*, p. 22.

[51]President's Commission for the Study of Ethical Problems in Medicine and Biomedical and Behavioral Research (1983) *Deciding to*

Forego Life-Sustaining Treatment. (US Government Printing Office, Washington, DC), pp. 82–90.

[52]Cited in President's Commission, p. 85, n. 122 (italics added).

[53]Lifton, p. 62.

[54]*Ibid.*

[55]Pence, G. E. (1988) Do not go slowly into that dark night: Mercy killing in Holland. *Am. J. Med.* **84,** p. 141.

[56]McCullogh, L., cited in Lamb, p. 29.

[57]Weisbard, A. J. and Siegler, M (1989) On killing patients with kindness: An appeal for caution, in *Ethical Issues in Modern Medicine,* 3rd ed. (Arras, J. D. and Rhoden, N. K., eds.), Mayfield Publishing, Mountain View, CA, p. 218.

[58]Callahan, D. (1987) *Setting Limits* (Simon and Schuster, New York), p. 179.

[59]Lamb, pp. 37–40.

[60]Weisbard and Siegler, pp. 218,219.

[61]Lifton, p. 418.

[62]Kronberg, p. 129.

[63]Neuhaus, p. 20 and passim.

[64]Weisbard and Siegler, p. 215.

[65]Noakes and Pridham, p. 1001.

[66]Rothenberg, L. S. (1987) *Guidelines on the Termination of Life-Sustaining Treatment and Care of the Dying.* The Hastings Center Appendix, p. 158.

[67]*Ibid.*

[68]*Guidelines,* p. 120.

[69]*Ibid.,* pp. 118–126.

[70]*Ibid.,* p. 120.

[71]*Ibid.,* p. 126.

[72]Noakes and Pridham, p. 997.

[73]Proctor (1988), p. 183.

Cranford Chapter

[1]Wanzer, S. H., Federman, D. D., Adelstein, S. J., et al. (1989) The physician's responsibility towards hopelessly ill patients. A second look. *N. Engl. J. Med.* **320,** 844–849.

[2]Wanzer, S. H., Adelstein, S. J, Cranford, R. E., et al. (1984) The physician's responsibility towards hopelessly ill patients. *New Engl. J. Med.* **310,** 955–959.

[3]The President's Commission for the Study of Ethical Problems in Medicine and Biomedical and Behavioral Research (1983) *Decid-*

ing to Forego Life-Sustaining Treatment. (US Government Printing Office, Washington, DC).

4Rothenberg, L. S. (1987) *Guidelines on the Termination of Life-Sustaining Treatment and the Care of the Dying. The Hastings Center.*

5Gaylin, W., Kass, L. R., Pellegrino, E. D., and Siegler, M. (1988)
Doctors must not kill. *JAMA* **259;14,** 2139–2140.

6Anonymous (1988) It's over Debbie. *JAMA* **259;2,** p. 272.

7Vaux, K. L. (1988) Debbie's dying: Mercy killing and the good death.
JAMA **259;14,** 2140,2141.

8Lundberg, G. D. (1988) 'It's Over Debbie' and euthanasia debate.
JAMA **259;14,** 2142,2143.

9Letters to the Editor, (1988) *JAMA* **259;14,** 2094–2098.

10Lifton, R. J. (1986) *The Nazi Doctors: Medical Killing and the Psychology of Genocide* (Basic Books, New York, NY).

11Proctor, R. N. (1988) *Racial Hygiene: Medicine Under the Nazis*
(Harvard University Press, Cambridge, MA).

12Admiraal, P. V. (1986) Euthanasia applied at a general hospital.
Euthanasia Rev. **1;2,** 97–107.

13Pence, G. E. (1988) Do not go slowly into that dark night: Mercy
killing in Holland. *Am. J. Med.* **84,** 139–141.

14Central Committee of the Royal Dutch Medical Association. (1984)
Vision on euthanasia. *Med. Contact.* **39,** 990–998.

15Final Report of the Netherland State Commission on Euthanasia:
An English Summary (1987) *Bioethics* 163–174.

16Kuhse, H. (1987) Voluntary euthanasia in the Netherlands. *Med.
J. Australia* **147,** 394–396.

17Gevers, J. K. M. (1987) Legal developments concerning active euthanasia on request in the Netherlands. *Bioethics* **1;2,** 156–162.

18Alexander, L. (1949) Medical science under dictatorship. *N. Engl.
J. Med.* **241,** 39–47.

Neuhaus Chapter

1Bopp, J. and Burtchaell, J. (1989) Fetal tissue transplantation: The
fetus as medical commodity. *This World: A J. Religion and Public
Life.* The Elie Wiesel quote appears in that article. For a thorough
documentation of analogies between the Holocaust and current
debates, *see* "Die Buben Sind Unser Unglueck" in Burtchaell, J.
(1982) *Rachel Weeping* (Harper & Row).

2Fackenheim, E. L. (1982) *To Mend the World* (Schocken Books).

3Oliner, S. and Oliner, P. (1988) *The Altruistic Personality* (Basic
Books, New York).

[4]Kass, L. R. (1985) Is there a medical ethic?: The Hippocratic Oath and the sources of ethical medicine, in *Toward a More Natural Science* (The Free Press); also, Kass, L. R. (1989) Why doctors must not kill. *The Public Interest*.

[5]Lasch, C. (1989) Engineering the good life. *This World*.

[6]Grobstein, C. (1989) *Science and the Unborn* (Basic Books, New York). For a more extended critique of Grobstein, *see* Neuhaus, (1989) After Roe v. Wade. *Commentary*. A more comprehensive discussion of current developments in bioethics is Neuhaus, (1988) The return of eugenics. *Commentary*. Also, *Guaranteeing the Good Life*, edited by Neuhaus, forthcoming from Eerdmans Publishing.

Katz Chapter

[1](1946–1949)*Trials of War Criminals Before the Nuremberg Military Tribunals Under Control Council Law No. 10,* vol. 1 (US Government Printing Office, Washington, DC), 39.

[2]*Ibid.*, p. 38.

[3]Katz, J. (1972) *Experimentation with Human Beings* (Russell Sage Foundation, New York), 1.

[4]Cahn, E. (1964) Drug experiments and the public conscience, in *Drugs in Our Society* (Talalay, P., ed.), Johns Hopkins Press, Baltimore, MD, p. 255.

[5]Veressayev, V. (1916) *The Memoirs of a Physician* (Linde, S., trans.), Alfred A. Knopf, New York, pp. 332–366. Reprinted in *Experimentation with Human Beings,* 284–291.

[6]V. Hubbenet, H. (1986) Observations and experiments in syphilis, *Medical-Military J.* part 77, p. 423.

[7]The American Humane Association (1901) *Concerning Human Vivisection—A Controversy*.

[8]Prinzmetal M. (1965) On the Humane Treatment of Charity Patients. *Medical Tribune,* 15.

[9]*Trials of War Criminals,* 92–198.

[10]Prinzmetal, M. (1965) On the humane treatment of charity patients. *Medical Tribune* **6,** 15.

[11]*Trials of War Criminals,* pp. 418–494.

[12]*Ibid.*, p. 73.

[13]*Ibid.*, pp. 477–484.

[14]*Ibid.*, vol. II 86.

[15]Beecher, H. K. (1966) Ethics and clinical research, *N. Engl. J. Med.* **274,** 1354–1360.

[16]Reprinted in *Experimentation with Human Beings,* 9–65.

[17]Final Report of the Tuskegee Syphilis Study Ad Hoc Advisory Panel. US Department of Health, Education and Welfare 1–47 (1973).

[18]*Ibid.*, pp. 14,15.

[19]Reprinted in *Experimentation with Human Beings*, 311.

[20]*Ibid.*

[21]Lifton, R. J. (1986) *The Nazi Doctors–Medical Killing and the Psychology of Genocide* (Basic Books, New York). The author offers many more reasons for the conduct of the Nazi physicians. I am indebted in this section to the account he has given of the Auschwitz experiments.

[22]*Ibid.*, p. 435.

[23]*Ibid.*, pp. 16,17.

[24]*Ibid.*, p. 16.

[25]*Ibid.*, p. 17.

[26]Katz, J. (1986) *The Silent World of Doctor and Patient* (The Free Press, New York).

[27]*The Nazi Doctors*, 208.

[28]Milgram, S. (1976) *Obedience to Authority* (Harper & Row, New York).

[29]*The Nazi Doctors*, 15,16.

[30]US Atomic Energy Commission, In the Matter of J. Robert Oppenheimer, *Transcript of Hearing Before Personnel Security Board.* Washington, DC: US Government Printing Office, pp. 249–251 (1954) [Hereafter: *Atomic Energy Commission*]

[31]Mazzeo, J. A. (1967) *The Design of Life* (Pantheon Books, New York).

[32]Malcolm, J. (1987, March 13) The journalist and the murderer. *The New Yorker,* pp. 38–73.

[33]Katz, J. (1986) *The Silent World* (The Free Press, New York), paperback ed.

[34]Sun, M. (1988) EPA ban use of Nazi data. *Science* **240**, p. 21.

[35]*The New York Times* 1 (23 March 1988).

[36]Freud, S. (1961) Civilization and its discontents, in *The Standard Edition of the Complete Psychological Works of Sigmund Freud.* **21**, 114.

[37]Katz, J. (1987) The regulation of human experimentation in the United States—A personal odyssey. *IRB* **9**, p. 6.

[38]Cahn, E. (1964) Drug experiments and the public conscience, in *Drugs in our Society* (Talalay, P. ed.), Johns Hopkins Press, Baltimore, MD, p. 260.

[39]*Atomic Energy Commission*, 251.

Seidelman Chapter

[1]Lifton, R. J. (1986) *The Nazi Doctors: Medical Killing and the Psychology of Genocide* (Basic Books, New York).

[2]Müller-Hill, B. (1988) *Murderous Science* (Oxford University Press, Oxford, UK).

[3]Mitscherlich, A. and Mielke, F. (1949) *Doctors of Infamy: The Story of the Nazi Medical Crimes* (Schuman, New York).

[4]*Ibid.*

[5]Mosse, G. L. (1978) *Toward the Final Solution. A History of European Racism* (Harper Colophon, New York).

[6]Schwartz, H. (1980) A person is a person and a shpos is not. *Man and Med.* **5**, 226–228.

[7]Shem, A. (1978) *The House of God* (Dell, New York).

[8]*Ibid.*

[9]Marrus, M. R. and Paxton, R. O. (1981) *Vichy France and the Jews* (Basic Books, New York).

[10]Pearle, K. M. (1981) Preventive medicine: The refugee physician and the New York medical community 1933–1945. Leibrief, S. and Tennstedt, F., eds., *Working Papers on Blocked Alternatives in the Health Policy System No. 11.* Research Center on Social Conditions, Social Movements and Social Policy at the University of Bremen, Bremen.

[11]Kohler, E. D. (1986) Between Dr. Pinkham's Dilemma and Dr. Mumey's Jerusalem: German Jewish Physicians in California and Colorado. Unpublished paper presented at German Studies Association Annual Meeting. Albuquerque, NM.

[12]Friedman, M. (1962) *Capitalism and Freedom* (University of Chicago Press, Chicago, IL).

[13]Blakeney, M. (1985) *Australia and the Jewish Refugees 1933–1948* (Croom Helm, Sydney).

[14]Government of Palestine. Annual Report of the Department of Health for the Year 1935.

[15]Medical Practitioners (Amendment) Ordinance, No. 44 of 1935. An Ordinance to Amend the Medical Practitioners Ordinance, 1928. 30th October, 1935. Israel State Archives, Record Group 2 M/74/35.

[16](1935, July 25) *Palestine Post*, p. 1.

[17](1935, July 29) Editorial. *Palestine Post*, p. 4.

[18]Hanauske-Abel, H. (1986) From nazi holocaust to nuclear holocaust: A lesson to learn? *Lancet* **2**, 271–273.

[19]Stock, U. (1987) Deutsche Ärzte und die Vergangenheit. *Die Zeit.* 56.

[20]Flexner, A. (1940) *I Remember* (Simon and Shuster, New York).

[21]Proctor R. (1988) *Racial Hygiene: Medicine Under the Nazis* (Harvard, Cambridge, MA).

[22]Dickman, S. (1989) Scandal over Nazi victims' corpses rocks universities. *Nature* **337**, p. 195.

[23]Dickman, S. (1989) Brain sections to be buried. *Nature* **339**, p. 498.

[24]Bogerts, B. (1988) The brains of the Vogt collection. *Arch. Gen. Psychiatry* **45,** p. 774.

[25]Gershon, E. S. and Hoehe, M. R. (1988) Comment: On the deaths of Ernst and Klaus H. *Arch. Gen. Psychiatry* **45,** 774,775.

[26]Rüdin, E. (1916) *Zur Verebung und Neuentstehung der Dementia praecox.* (Springer, Berlin).

[27]Wistrich, R. (1982) *Who's Who in the Third Reich* (Weidenfeld and Nicholson, London).

[28]Stern, K. (1951) *The Pillar of Fire* (Harcourt-Brace, New York).

[29]Sherrinton, R., Brynjolfsson, J., Petursson, H., Potter, M., Dudleston, K., Barraclough, B., Wasmuth, J., Dobbs M., and Gurling H. (1988) *Nature* **336,** 164–167.

[30]Seidelman, W. (1989) Lessons from eugenic history. *Nature* **337,** p. 300.

[31]Von Verschuer, O. (1939) Twin research from the time of Francis Galton to the present day. *Proc. R. Soc. London* **128,** 62–81.

[32]Gedda L. (1956) Un maestro e un esempio. *Acta Genet. Med. Gemellol. (Roma).* Suppl. Primum. **5,** 241–248.

[33]Müller-Hill, B. (1987) Genetics after Auschwitz. *Holocaust Genocide Stud.* **2,** 3–20.

[34]*Ibid.*

[35]Nyiszli, M. (1960) *Auschwitz* (Fawcett, New York).

[36]Kater, M. H. (1987) The burden of the past: Problems of a modern historiography of physicians and medicine in Nazi Germany. *German Stud. Rev.* **10,** 31–57.

[37]*Ibid.*

[38]Seidelman, W. (1988) Mengele medicus: Medicine's nazi heritage. *Milbank Q.* **66,** 221–239.

[39]Angel, M. D. (1980) *The Jews of Rhodes* (Sepher-Hermon, New York).

Segal Chapter

[1]Segal, N. L. (1989) Twin survivors of Auschwitz-Birkenau: Behavioral, medical and social issues. *Proceedings from Remembering for the Future* (Pergamon Press, Oxford, UK), pp. 2288–2298.

[2]Segal, N. L. (1990) The importance of twin studies for individual differences research. *J. Couns. Dev.* **68,** 612–622.

[3]Posner, G. L. and Ware, J. J. (1986) *Mengele: The Complete Story* (McGraw-Hill, New York).

[4]Nyiszli, M. (1960) *Auschwitz: A Doctor's Eyewitness Account* (Kremer, T. and Seaver, R., trans.), Fawcett Crest, New York.

[5]I was present at both the reunion at Auschwitz-Birkenau and the hearing at Yad VaShem.

[6]Lifton, R. J. (1982) Medicalized killing in Auschwitz. *Psychiatry* **45**, 283–297.

[7]Lifton, R. J. (1986) *The Nazi Doctors* (Basic Books, New York).

[8]Greulich, W. W. (1934) Heredity in human twinning. A*m. J. Phys. Anthr.* **19**, 391–431.

[9]Members of the panel included Gideon Hausner, Chairman of the Panel and Chief Prosecutor at the Eichmann Trial; Simon Wiesenthal, Director of the Documentation Center of the Federation of Jewish Victims of the Nazi Regime, Vienna, Austria; Telford Taylor, Prosecutor at the Nuremberg Trials, Arno Motulsky, Professor of Genetics at the University of Washington in Seattle, WA; Yehuda Bauer, Professor of History at the Hebrew University in Jerusalem, Israel; Zvi Terlo, Attorney and Former Head of the Israeli Ministry of Justice; and Rafi Eitan, Former Advisor to the Israeli Government on Terrorism. Expert opinion was provided by a psychiatrist, the late Professor Shamai Davidson from Bar-Ilan University in Israel.

[10]Hausner, G., Bauer, Y., Eitan, R., Motulsky, A., Taylor, T., Terlo, Z., and Wiesenthal, S. (1985) *The International Commission of Inquiry Into Josef Mengele's Crimes Resolutions.* Yad VaShem, Jerusalem.

[11]Lykken, D. T. (1978) The diagnosis of zygusity in twins. *Behav. Genet.* **8**, 437–473.

[12]Segal, N. L. (1984) Zygusity testing: Laboratory and the investigator's judgment. *Acta Genet. Med. et Gemellol.* **33**, 515–521.

[13]de Azevedo, A. (1944) Uber die erblichkeit der quantitat der blutgruppensubstanzen. *Der Erbarzt.* **12**, 85–90.

[14]The Kaiser-Wilhelm Institute in Berlin received data and specimens collected by Mengele at Auschwitz-Birkenau. The director at that time was Otmar F. Von Verschuer, who obtained research funding for Mengele's experiments.

[15]Segal, N. L. (1985) Holocaust twins: Their special bond. *Psychol. Today* **19**, 52–58.

[16]Segal, N. L. (1988) Cooperation, competition, and altruism in human twinships: A sociobiological approach, in *Sociobiological Perspectives on Human Development* (MacDonald, K. B., ed.), Springer-Verlag, New York, pp. 168–206.

[17]Soble, R. (1989, Mar. 3). U.S. secrecy keeps cloud of doubt over Mengele death. *Los Angeles Times.*

[18]Wiesenthal, S. (1989) Doubts about Mengele's death. *Dokumentationszentrum, Bull.* **29**, 1,2.

[19]Becker, B. (1988) Comment: On the deaths of Ernst and Klaus H. *Arch. Gen. Psychiatry* **45**, p. 775.

[20]Bogerts, B. (1988) The brains of the Vogt collection. *Arch. Gen. Psychiatry* **45**, p. 774.

[21]Gershon, E. S. and Hoehe, M. R. (1988) Comment: On the deaths of Ernst and Klaus H. *Arch. Gen. Psychiatry* **45,** 775,776.

[22]Bogerts, B., Meertz, E., and Schoenfeld-Bausch, R. (1985) Basal ganglia and limbic system pathology in schizophrenia: A morphometric study of brain volume and shrinkage. *Arch. Gen. Psych.* **42,** 784–791.

Annas Chapter

[1]Portions of this section are adapted from Annas, G. J. (1989) Who's afraid of the human genome? *Hastings Cent. Rep.* 19–21.

[2]Editorial (1989, March 16) Chromosome cartography. *Wall Street Journal* p. A16 (emphasis added).

[3]See Annas, G. J. and Elias, S., eds. (1992) *Gene Mapping: Using Law and Ethics as Guidelines* (Oxford University Press, New York).

[4]Jaroff, L. (1989, March 20) The gene hunt. *Time* pp. 62–67.

[5]Watson, J. (1990) The human genome project: Past, present, and future. *Science* **248**, p. 44.

[6]Watson, J. (1968) *The Double Helix* (Macmillan, New York), p. xi.

[7]Rhodes, R. (1986) *The Making of the Atomic Bomb* (Simon & Schuster, New York), p. 761 (emphasis supplied).

[8]McDougall, W. (1985) *The Heavens and the Earth* (Basic Books, New York), p. 413.

[9]Portions of this section are adapted from Annas, G. J. (1990) Mapping the human genome and the meaning of monster mythology. *Emory Law J.* pp. 629–664.

[10]See, e.g., Macklin, R. (1986) Mapping the human genome: Problems of privacy and free choice, in *Genetics and the Law III* (Milunsky, A. and Annas, G. J., eds.), Plenum, New York, pp. 107–114.

[11]Proctor, R. N. (1988) *Racial Hygiene* (Harvard University Press, Cambridge, MA).

[12]*Buck v. Bell,* 274 U.S. 200, 207 (1927).

[13]US Congress, Office of Technology Assessment (1988) *Mapping Our Genes,* p. 84.

[14]*Ibid.* (emphasis added)

[15]Posner, G. L. and Ware, J. (1986) *Mengele: The Complete Story* (McGraw Hill, New York).

[16]*Ibid.*

[17]Lifton, R. J. (1986) *The Nazi Doctors* (Basic Books, New York).

[18]Müller Hill, B. (1987) Genetics after Auschwitz. *Holocaust and Genocide Stud.* **2**, 3–20.

[19]*Ibid.*

[20]Seidelman, W. E. (1988) Mengele medicus: Medicine's nazi heritage. *Milbank Mem. Q.* **66**, 221–239.

[21]McKusick, V. A. (1982) The human genome through the eyes of a clinical geneticist. *Cytogent. Cell Genet.* **32**, 7–23. Von Verschuer's work, along with that of almost 40,000 other authors, is also in all eight editions of Victor McKusick's classic work, *Medelian Inheritance in Man: Catalogs of Autosomal Dominant, Autosomal Recessive and X-Linked Phenotypes* (Johns Hopkins University Press, Baltimore, MD) The 8th edition, for example, cites Verschuer's 1938 article on dwarfism (twice), and his 1958 text on human genetics (Lehrbuch de Humanaenetik)(twice).

[22]The concept of "a species mentality" is discussed at some length in Lifton, R. J. and Markusen, E. (1990) *The Genocidal Mentality: Nazi Holocaust and Nuclear Threat* (Basic Books, New York), pp. 255–279.

[23]Roberts, L. (1988) Carving up the human genome. *Science* p. 1244.

[24]Havel, V. (1984) Politics and Conscience, an address sent by Havel to the University of Toulouse on the occasion of his being awarded an honorary doctorate, in *Living in Truth* (Vladislav, J., ed.), Faber & Faber, London.

[25]*Ibid.*

[26](1990, Feb. 22) Excerpts from Czech Chief's Address to Congress, *NY Times*, A14.

[27]Lifton and Markusen, *supra* note 22 at 259.

Index